Promoting Acceptance of Children with Disabilities: *From Tolerance to Inclusion*

by P. Ann MacCuspie, Ph.D.

APSEA

Atlantic Provinces Special Education Authority
Halifax, Nova Scotia, Canada

ISBN 0-9680388-0-8
Printed by Halcraft Printers Inc., Halifax, Nova Scotia
Design: Janet Milbury

This book is for sale from:

APSEA

Atlantic Provinces Special Education Authority
BOOK ORDERS
5940 South Street, Halifax,
Nova Scotia, Canada B3H 1S6
Tel: (902) 424-8500
Fax: (902) 424-0543

Contents

Foreword

Promoting Acceptance of Children with Disabilities: From Tolerance to Inclusion is an important book. Although social and educational policies of inclusion are widely accepted in North America, they cannot be implemented without changes to many aspects of school practice. Ann MacCuspie's thoughtful study of the social lives of children with visual impairments in public schools uncovers many of the obstacles to social integration.

The struggles of children who are different or disabled to gain peer acceptance and approval are sometimes overwhelming. Barriers to participation are created when children are defined by their disabilities. Negative attitudes and lowered expectations create conditions for social isolation.

Children reflect the attitudes of the society in which they live. Myths, misinformation, fear, and pity lead to stereotypic images of children with visual problems. These images distort perceptions and prevent children from being viewed as individuals with abilities as well as disabilities. The book carefully examines the complexities of peer group acceptance, uncovers sources of confusion, and most importantly, it illustrates ways of creating social climates where individual children, disabled or not, can experience being valued and accepted for themselves.

Including children with disabilities in public education is widely accepted in educational jurisdictions all over North America. The movement to end segregated education gathered steam in the wake of the civil rights movement and was proclaimed educational policy in Canada and the United States. It is interesting to note that the history of the blindness field records a dynamic movement from segregation to integration. Blind people themselves have been the most determined, the most outspoken, and the most effective advocates of integration. Leaders in the blindness field pushed hard for social integration and proclaimed that "segregation in school leads to segregation in life."

The school is the child's link with his or her community. The classroom is the arena for making friends and understanding the world of peers. Children learn to use a wide range of strategies to gain acceptance and establish their identities among their peers. Feelings of belonging and recognition are achieved along with experience initiating interactions and becoming part of the peer group. To be fully accepted involves understanding peer group values and acquiring a range of social skills.

Visual impairments impose limitations on the ease with which children acquire information about their peers, their dress, their activities, and the intricacies of their play. Dr. MacCuspie succeeds in providing a sensitive examination of the intricacies of peer group interactions and her book contains many suggestions for parents, educators, and administrators.

The specialized teaching, (e.g., instruction in braille and orientation and mobility), the special equipment used (e.g., magnifiers and braillers), and the use of adapted teaching materials may serve to further isolate the child and give him or her too high a profile in the classroom. This book offers valuable discussion about providing for special needs in ways that promote understanding and acceptance in the classroom.

Ann MacCuspie also explores the contradictions inherent in some school practices. While acceptance and honoring of differences among students is proclaimed, reward and recognition may be given only to high academic achievers. The resulting competition generated may work against the child with a disability as well as other children who struggle with being different. Children who learn in a different way, or use different materials may be excluded and not expected to participate.

One of the greatest benefits of inclusion or integrated education is the fostering of positive social attitudes and respect for differences. Children learn to care about one another and cooperate in social environments where individual differences are valued and acknowledged. One of the greatest values of integrated education is the opportunities it provides for every child to feel valued and contribute to the self respect of other children. Dr. MacCuspie raises the issue of the school's responsibility to social as well as cognitive development. This issue is a central concern of parents and educators and this book confronts the issue with honesty and candor. The many suggestions provided in ***Promoting Acceptance of Children with Disabilities: From Tolerance to Inclusion*** can make the school experience richer for all children. This book is a valuable contribution to making integration and inclusion a reality for all children.

Sally Rogow, Ed.D.
Professor Emerita
University of British Columbia

Preface

*Of all the blessings that time and earth bestow, there is none so precious as one true friend.**

The social interaction of children with a visual impairment has intrigued me since my first encounter with a group of children from the Halifax School for the Blind. As a volunteer helping in a swimming program for elementary level children, I was surprised to observe how similar their interactions were to those of sighted children of the same age. The next year, while studying for my Masters in Education of the Visually Impaired, I lived at Perkins School for the Blind in a residence with twenty-nine boys ranging from nine to thirteen years of age. As a teacher-trainee, I was immersed in the social world of these delightful individuals. Many hours were spent both playing with them and observing them as they participated in residence, school, and recreational activities. Throughout all these experiences, I paid particular attention to the interactions among these children, how their friendships developed, the factors which tended to bring some children together and those that excluded others.

The social life of children in a residential setting proved intriguing. I have particularly vivid memories of the game with the "outsiders." From time to time, the boys would gather near the fence separating the school grounds from the residential neighbourhood in which it was located. From the safety of their fenced-in area, they would exchange insults and sometimes hurled objects (e.g., apples, snowballs, rocks) at some of the neighbourhood children (i.e., "the outsiders").

Several years later, while teaching at the Halifax School for the Blind in Nova Scotia, I was interested to observe that a similar game with the "outsiders" was well established. A second enlightening experience in relation to the social interaction between children who were visually impaired and their fully sighted peers occurred one weekend when a ten year old boy with low vision accompanied me to my parent's home for the Easter weekend. Having a younger brother of the same age, I anticipated they would play together and have lots of things in common. The weekend, although an enjoyable outing for the student from the school, was a very stressful one for my brother. Expressions of confusion and hesitation were routinely evident as he interacted with the boy who was visually impaired. Now, as an adult, my brother recalls the discomfort created by not knowing if he should respond to the other boy's

* Used with permission and published by Celex Group, Inc./Celebrating Excellance, all rights reserved.

invitation to wrestle, how to make eye contact with one whose eyes were constantly in motion, and how to choose activities which would be appropriate for this new acquaintance. Obviously, some formal intervention prior to the visit could have alleviated some of the uneasiness experienced by my brother as well as the restraint on spontaneous interaction between the two boys.

Later in my teaching career, I became involved in a pilot project designed to integrate a group of students who were visually impaired into a local elementary school near the Halifax School for the Blind. While enthusiastically announcing this exciting project to the Grade IV students who were to be integrated the next year, I was overwhelmed when three of the ten children began to cry. Through discussion and attentive listening it became evident that these children had many fears and concerns about the prospect of daily interaction with "sighted kids." Although we were able to alleviate much of their distress through exchange visits with their new schoolmates, role-playing, and discussion groups, it was evident following the first year of the project that all ten children had remained "on the fringe" of social life in the public school setting.

The integration of students with a visual impairment into regular classrooms continued to be promoted throughout Canada and the United States during the next few decades. In Atlantic Canada, as we gained more experience with the process of integration and had opportunities to speak with teachers and parents of children with a visual impairment, a common concern became apparent — these children were not experiencing the same level of social acceptance as the majority of their fully sighted classmates. Itinerant teachers for the visually impaired and parents of the integrated students routinely reported these children had few "real friends."

The reasons behind these difficulties with social integration tormented me. Why was this happening? From my adult perspective, these children had much to offer a friend. Many were good students, had delightful personalities, dressed appropriately, shared interests common to their age group, yet, they struggled with social acceptance by their peers. It was the search for a clearer understanding of the complex issues involved in the social acceptance of children who are different which led me to pursue research in this area. This book is the end product of much observation, research, interviewing, and analyzing to better understand the world of children and their friendships. Still, it is only a beginning. As educators and parents consider some of the ideas and implement some of the suggestions contained in this book, new understanding and strategies will emerge. Individuals will discover better ways to enhance the social acceptance of a given child in a particular situation. Schools will become more adept at welcoming and including a population characterized by diversity. The goal of the book is to contribute to the understanding that will prompt action to make these things happen.

This book is divided into three sections. Section I presents an introduction to the issues associated with the social integration of children with a visual impairment. In Chapter 1, concepts relevant to integration and the complex variables inherent in stereotypes, social relationships, and acceptance by others are considered. A general overview of social development is provided in Chapter 2. The interactions of children and youth, the nature of their friendships, and the findings of research on the social acceptance of children with disabilities are reviewed. In the final chapter of this section, Chapter 3, information on visual impairment and factors influencing the social interaction and acceptance of individuals with a visual impairment are presented.

Section II of the book is devoted to a report on a qualitative research study which examined the social integration of five children who were visually impaired and who were integrated in regular classrooms at the elementary school level. In Chapter 4, findings of the research relevant to pupil culture and the role it played in the acceptance of those perceived to be different are examined. The cultural assumptions associated with adults participating in the school environment and those relevant to social integration are analyzed in Chapter 5. In Chapter 6, the risks to the development of positive self-esteem in children with a visual impairment who are integrated without appropriate intervention to encourage positive interaction with peers are discussed.

In the final section of the book, specific suggestions and recommendations to enhance the social acceptance and interaction of students with disabilities who are integrated in our schools are addressed. The role of a collaborative team in planning for social integration is outlined in Chapter 7. In addition to general suggestions, specific suggestions for teachers, parents, and teachers of the visually impaired are provided. In the final chapter, controversial issues associated with the social integration in the school environment are considered. Issues such as the role of the teacher assistant and the responsibility of classroom teachers to implement social skills training are discussed. The book contains four appendices which provide information about resources and materials to assist parents and educators in addressing the social integration of students with a disability as well as checklists which can be used to guide the collaborative team in their planning for the inclusion of all students.

Acknowledgements

I am indebted to the many people who assisted in the development of this book and the research on which it is based. I am especially grateful to the five students with a visual impairment and their classmates who shared their beliefs about friendship and their perceptions on the world, i.e., the world of children. To the teachers, principals, parents of the five children with a visual impairment, and the itinerant teachers for the visually impaired, I acknowledge their contribution of opinions, emotions and ideas. They permitted access to the social world of the children and shared their perceptions of the acceptance and interaction of these students.

A very special expression of gratitude is extended to Dr. Jennifer Hill, a good friend, who contributed her time to review and proofread the book. Also, to Mr. Daniel Harmer, former Director of the Atlantic Provinces Special Education Authority Resource Centre for the Visually Impaired, I acknowledge the valuable insights and thought provoking discussions shared after reading the original research. To Alma Boutilier, a colleague and adept proofreader, I extend a heartfelt thank you for her willingness to volunteer her skills and her support. I feel honoured that a renown educator of children with a visual impairment, Dr. Sally Rogow, has written the forward for my book and am grateful for her contribution.

Finally, I wish to express my appreciation to my husband Ormand, who was always a source of encouragement and motivation, and to my daughter Jillian, who enthusiastically shared her insights and perspectives on childhood friendships.

Section I

Social Integration of Children with a Visual Impairment

1

Integration and Social Acceptance - Getting It into Perspective

Introduction

Integration, the education of children with disabilities in the regular classroom, is a complex practice. As educators experiment with the implementation of integration, there are different emphasis and varied concerns from all participants involved. There are parents' concerns about the child's social well-being and the amount of instruction that will be provided. Regular classroom teachers have concerns about the special needs of the child with a disability and the practicality of meeting such needs simultaneously with those of the other twenty-five to thirty-five students in the classroom. There are specialist teachers' concerns about ensuring the child receives the compensatory skills required to benefit from the learning environment in the regular class. From an administrator's perspective, there are concerns about safety, building access, teacher training, teacher stress, and the availability of essential funding and resources. The parents of other children in the classroom have concerns about how much of the classroom teacher's time will be devoted primarily to the student with the disability and the effect of this on the learning of the other children. The classmates, themselves, may have concerns about how to interact with a student with a disability. Finally, there are the concerns of the child with a disability about being accepted by peers. Inherent in all of the above, of course, are the philosophical issues associated with prejudice, stigma, and the positive acceptance of difference in our schools.

Teachers face an intriguing challenge as they prepare to deal with the social integration of children with disabilities who are enrolled in their classrooms. Integration involves a multitude of interrelated issues such as the provision of appropriate programming, the level of teacher expertise and cooperation, the influence of cultural beliefs and attitudes, the promotion of social relationships, and the availability of support services. By developing an overview of the complexities associated with integration, this complex concept can be brought more clearly into perspective. As parents and educators begin to plan for the social acceptance of students with disabilities, the many beliefs and issues which are intricately associated with or influenced by integration must first be acknowledged and understood. These include the concept of integration and its intended goals and practices, the attitudes associated with those who are disabled and their inclusion in society, and finally, the types of social relationships which are characteristic of school-age children and the importance of peer acceptance. Since collaboration among parents, educators and students is an essential component of successful integration, the challenge integration presents must be approached with essential information, insight, and above all, open-mindedness.

Because integration is such a complex concept, it is tremendously vulnerable to misinterpretation and the implementation of inappropriate practices and programs. Yet, integration holds tremendous potential to enhance both the educational and social-emotional development of children with disabilities. Within an inclusive school environment, both the individual learning needs of a given child and the importance of social relationships are considered when programs are planned and implemented. As the twenty-first century approaches, the degree to which integration is successful may be one measure of the extent to which education has met the individual and societal goals of this generation.

Currently, however, there are varied perspectives and beliefs among those working to promote the integration of students with disabilities and among those who are reluctant to embrace this practice. Social and psychological aspects of the educational setting such as stigma, stereotype, and attitude play a prominent role in how effectively integration is implemented and accommodated in a given school. For parents it can be painful to witness their child's social isolation when peer acceptance is not spontaneous. It is stressful to devote considerable effort to the ongoing advocacy required to ensure their child has the opportunity to receive an appropriate education. Parents struggle with efforts to be supportive without being overprotective and with having to deal with prejudice through understanding rather than with anger. Many organizational variables such as the quality of leadership, teacher empathy and expertise, and administrative flexibility affect the success of the integration process. A placement which works marvellously one year can be a traumatic failure the next year if the teacher does not promote the positive acceptance of difference or if the necessary support services are not made available.

Finally, it is important to understand the types of relationships children are forming at various times in their development and at different stages in their schooling experience. Just as social development has a cognitive component which will affect the types of relationships children develop, integration has a cultural aspect which will influence peer acceptance and interaction. Social and cultural variables will require educators and parents to observe, evaluate and modify the learning environments created for school children. Most importantly, they must routinely assess the perceptions of students with disabilities and those of their peers to ensure their experiences with integration are the positive ones which have been envisioned.

The Concept of Integration

Philosophies and practices associated with the education of children with disabilities in Canada have undergone considerable change during the last two decades. Children who were once believed to be uneducable and deprived of any formal educational experience are now considered to have the right to appropriate educational opportunities (MacKay, 1986). Students with a visual impairment who were often segregated in private schools for the duration of their school years may now attend their local public schools. In most cases they are enrolled in the regular classroom with peers who are fully sighted.

The concept of mainstreaming has been a guiding force in this change in educational placement for students who have a visual impairment. It originated from the philosophical belief called normalization, which contends that regardless of the severity or type of impairment the individual should live and be educated in as normal an environment as possible (Winzer, 1990). First implemented in the Scandinavian countries, the normalization movement focused on deinstitutionalization of those with an intellectual disability. Inherent in the movement of children and adults from institutions was the promotion of the goal of normal family and community life for those with disabilities, regardless of the type or severity of the disability (Wolfensberger, 1972). Opposed to life-long institutionalization, the concept of normalization was intended to offer "the handicapped the chance of a normal life routine, normal developmental experiences, independent choices, and the right to live, work, and play in normal surroundings" (Winzer, Rogow & David, 1987, p. 13).

In the United States, the extension of the principles of normalization to the educational setting in the 1970s became known as mainstreaming (Reynolds, 1976). Given an appropriate educational placement in a regular classroom, a student with a disability is expected to benefit from exposure to "normal" role models, opportunities to socialize with peers who are not nondisabled and learning experiences considered essential for all children. From a more theoretical perspective, mainstreaming was viewed as an effort to decrease the isolation of children with impairments confined to residential settings. Society would be exposed to those with disabilities thereby decreasing the stigma of labels such as "blind" or "deaf". Mainstreaming was also viewed as an opportunity to improve the educational opportunities for students with disabilities by shifting the emphasis from remediation based upon the student's impairment to a focus on specific, individual learning needs of the child (Barton & Tomlinson, 1981).

The concept of mainstreaming or integration, used interchangeably in this book, has been a source of much confusion as it has evolved and been implemented during the last three decades (Biklen, 1985; Gaylord-Ross, 1989). As early as 1974 in an article entitled "Will the Real 'Mainstreaming' Program Please Stand Up! (Or...Should Dunn Have Done It?)", Chaffin alerted educators to the diversity of programs alleged to be incorporating the philosophies and/or practices inherent in mainstreaming. Even within this early article the term "mainstreaming" was used interchangeably as both a philosophy and a practice.

As is common to many educational innovations, during the process of implementation the original essence of the concept may be changed to accommodate existing circumstances within a particular school or district. Factors such as the availability of trained personnel, resources, and funding have a significant effect upon the level of mainstreaming which evolves in a given case. For example, some students with disabilities are enrolled fulltime in the regular class; others may spend all or a certain percentage of their time in special classes within the public school. Some pupils receive individual instruction within the regular class; others are removed for special instruction. Some students have a student-assistant assigned to work directly with them; others have access to an assistant who has been assigned to help the classroom teacher. Finally, some pupils attend their neighbourhood school while others must travel to a district school designated for special programs. However, more important than the diversity of administrative arrangements as it relates to service delivery models is the emphasis programs place on acceptance and active participation of students with disabilities. Unfortunately, a program focus on peer acceptance and interaction appears to be as varied and diverse as are the service delivery models.

What Does Integration Mean?

Integration or mainstreaming refers to the process of educating children with disabilities with their peers who are not disabled in a public school setting. Gall (1987) suggests that there are three interdependent elements that must be considered in actualizing integration. The first, temporal integration, refers to the actual time spent in the regular classroom. A child must spend a significant portion of the day, at least fifty percent of the time, in the regular classroom. The second element, instructional integration, emphasizes the importance of having students with disabilities actively involved in the instructional activities in the classroom. This involvement might encompass adapted activities or completion of the same curriculum as other classmates. Finally, the third element, social integration, focuses on the interaction and acceptance of children with disabilities by their classmates. The interdependence of these three elements is crucial to the implementation of integration.

The individual needs of each child should be carefully considered as educational opportunities are created. For the majority of children with a disability, full integration in the public school system should be the norm. For some students with a disability, placement outside the regular classroom for some portion of the school day may be warranted for specific instructional needs. For example, students with a visual impairment need to learn compensatory skills such as those associated with orientation and mobility training or the use of special technology. For this instruction, removal from the classroom may be necessary. For a very few children who are disabled, a short-term segregated placement outside the public school system may be justified, if the return of the student to the public school setting as soon as feasible is explicit to the goal of this placement.

Integration needs to be viewed as an ongoing process in each classroom. Circumstances vary not just from year to year but from day to day. Some activities on a given day may not be appropriate for a child who is totally blind (e.g., the dodge ball game in physical education class). Obviously, there must be flexibility to accommodate the individual needs of the child as the day to day events unfold. As with any educational innovation, extensive preparation and planning precede the actual implementation of integration. Once initiated, the process should be closely monitored, evaluated, and adjusted to respond to the various aspects of a given school, its population, and most importantly, the needs of the integrated child and her/his family. Teachers, parents, administrators, and, when appropriate, classmates, and the student should work closely together to plan programs to meet the identified needs of the child with a disability. Such a "problem-solving attitude" is an essential feature of the integration process (Biklen, 1985). The provision of adequate resources; flexible programming options; interdisciplinary approaches to problem-solving; and prominent administrative, moral, and practical support characterize the real intent of integration, that is, the meaningful inclusion of children with disabilities in their homes, schools, and communities.

Just as the integration of children with disabilities requires significant changes in the regular classroom, it also demands an examination of the appropriateness of programs and services traditionally offered by special education staff (e.g., physiotherapy, speech therapy). Effective provision within the integrated setting will necessitate both innovative thinking and practices. Flexibility and teamwork, the hallmarks of successful integration programs, require parents and educators to consider the individual needs of children with disabilities at various times and stages of development in their school careers.

Inherent in the concept of integration is the restructuring of the existing educational system to better meet the needs of all students, not just those who can be categorized into a variety of existing classifications for children with impairments (Quintal, 1986; Sapon-Shevin, 1978). Proponents of restructuring have suggested the need for a merging of special and regular education –a merger that deletes ineffective educational practices and adopts those which promote better opportunities for all children. Such a merger incorporates "demonstrably effective practices from special, compensatory, and general education to establish a general education system that is more inclusive and that better serves all students" (Reynolds Wang, & Walberg, 1987, p. 394).

During the 1990s, inclusive education has become the term used to indicate the intended meaning of integration promoted by early advocates. The goals of inclusive education are:

> *to foster lifelong learning, provide educational quality and equity, facilitate independent learning and thinking, promote a school-home partnership, encourage living and learning in a community, and develop the academic and social competence of all students.*
> *(Andrews & Lupart, 1993, p. 5)*

Inclusive education demands that educators create a learning environment that values all students equally and reflects the heterogeneous nature of society in regular classrooms. Most importantly, it makes very explicit the responsibilities educators have to address both the academic and the social needs of students.

Hopefully, it is becoming apparent that philosophies such as integration or inclusion cannot be imposed upon the general education system and be expected to be successfully implemented without significant restructuring of the entire system. Those aspects of the regular education system which have posed the most serious barriers to full integration appear to be the same features responsible for the less than satisfactory performance of many children who are not disabled—aspects such as highly competitive classroom environments (Sapon-Shevin, 1978) and teaching to the needs of the average child.

If integration is to succeed, it must be considered as an effort to realize the positive acceptance of difference. Those who envisioned and promoted the concept of normalization, as extended to and developed in the public school system, have always intended that children with disabilities be accepted by their peers and that this acceptance be evidenced by regular spontaneous interaction with peers in both school and community activities (Gall, 1987; Quintal, 1986). Researchers (Sacks, Kekelis & Gaylord-Ross, 1992) have frequently documented an existing relationship between the level of social competence in childhood and the long-term emotional adjustment of individuals. Lack of acceptance by one's peers during the elementary school years is one of the very few facets of childhood functioning that consistently predicts behaviour problems or emotional disturbance in adolescence and adulthood (Hartup, 1984). Similarly, mental illness in adult life is often correlated with social isolation in childhood (Cowen, Pederson, Babigian, Izzo, & Trost, 1973). Therefore, if we are to ensure the intent of integration is realized, there is an urgent need to identify the specific socialization process experienced by children with disabilities and the type and level of interaction in their everyday lives which perpetuate or contribute to their exclusion from meaningful social relationships with their peers.

What Integration Should Not Mean

One of the unfortunate consequences of the integration movement for some children with disabilities has been the phasing out of, or limiting of access to, programs considered critical to the development of the student (e.g., instruction to develop independent living skills). Integration was not intended to diminish the learning opportunities or options available to children. On the contrary, it was intended to increase access to many new opportunities by having children both learn the special skills they require to compensate for their disability and have exposure to the world of "school" experienced by the majority of youth in our society.

A second negative consequence of integration may be the reduction in the availability of opportunities for children with disabilities to associate with peers who have similar disabilities. In some situations involvement of this kind is openly discouraged by both parents and educators. Yet, children who share a common disability, such as a visual impairment, frequently benefit from the opportunity to interact with peers encountering similar life experiences such as dealing with one's acceptance of being disabled, being the only student with a visual impairment in one's school, or being ineligible for a driver's license. In school districts where students with a visual impairment have been periodically brought together for instruction and interaction, tremendous social benefits and supportive relationships have evolved (MacCuspie, Harmer, McConnell, Fricker, & Johnson, 1993). These types of experiences are often critical to the child's development of self-concept and positive self-esteem. Social isolation in the mainstream was not anticipated by the proponents of integration. Yet, for many students with disabilities, social acceptance by their classroom peers appears to be one of the "missing links" in the integration process. Addressing this component of integration is, perhaps, the greatest challenge educators and parents will face.

Stigma, Stereotype, and Attitude

In attempting to identify and analyze the many complex factors inherent in integration, it is important to both acknowledge and address the role of attitudes. For the most part, our society holds negative attitudes toward those who are perceived to be different from the norm. This process should not create a sense of guilt, but rather should provide an awareness of how attitudes and beliefs evolve in our culture as well as how society chooses to deal with those involved. Such insight is critical to the modification of inaccurate or inappropriate beliefs and attitudes.

In the research literature on integration, the importance of a supportive and positive attitude by teachers, parents, and administrators has been well documented. Successful integration and social acceptance cannot be instituted by law nor by pressure from advocacy groups. In the final analysis, the positive attitude of informed classroom teachers and their willingness to promote and strive to achieve the benefits of integration will be the real determinants of success.

To understand how people develop beliefs and attitudes relevant to integration, it is helpful to understand the conceptual distinctions among the terms impairment, disability, and handicap. An impairment is a condition resulting from an anatomical or functional disorder. For example, a person who has permanent damage to the retina of the eye has a visual impairment. One who suffers significant brain damage as a result of a car accident or inherits a condition characterized by malfunctioning of specific areas of the brain has a neurological impairment. Thus, to indicate that an individual has an impairment is to assume the body is different in some anatomical or physiological way.

Disability reflects the consequence of an impairment. If, because of the presence of an impairment, an individual cannot complete a specific task or meet the expectations for a given role, task or activity, that person is said to have a disability (Nixon, 1991). A disability is not always evident in all situations. For example, a student who is blind and who is provided with a braille copy of the class handout is not disabled in relation to accessing the information on the handout or discussing the information with peers; however, if a braille copy of the handout is not provided, the student who is blind is then disabled if information on the handout is required for active participation or completion of a specific activity. Similarly, a person with a visual impairment who has learned to travel safely and efficiently using a white cane may become disabled if, for some reason, they are required to travel without the use of the cane. For many children with low vision, their first encounter with being disabled occurs when they enroll in school and have difficulty functioning in classrooms where their learning needs have not been identified and addressed.

The term handicapped is associated with a socially inferior status (Nixon, 1991). A handicap is the resulting disadvantages which occur when society does not adapt the physical or social environment to accommodate limitations created by an impairment but then places a negative value judgement on the impaired individual's social or moral worth. Students with disabilities are handicapped in an integrated school placement when they are placed in situations which compromise their value as students. For example, when the lack of brailled materials limits the student's meaningful participation in an activity and creates the belief that this student is either incapable or not worthy of inclusion, the student is handicapped. The critical recognition is that society has handicapped the student.

Cultural beliefs also influence the way society responds to those who have an impairment. In examining the way such beliefs guide behaviour, it is important to recognize how attitudes consciously and unconsciously evolve. Stereotypes are developed as one gathers, processes, and integrates knowledge. Allport (1958) has argued that the human mind creates and uses categories to sort and organize the extensive amount of information which is received each day. People have categories for such things as "good friends", "acquaintances", "appropriate behaviour", "inappropriate behaviour", "teachers", and "blind people." As categories are established, new and old information is gathered in classes and clusters which are used to guide our daily thinking and responses to our environment. For example, people have concepts and expectations associated with schools which guide responses to any newly presented information about schools. Therefore, if one attended a school in which all "slow learners" were enrolled in a special class in the basement of the school, one might be sceptical about the introduction of integration. It is important to note that it is just as simple to develop irrational categories as it is to create rational ones. This being the case, an individual might have limited options in her/his category of "jobs for people who are blind." Therefore, upon meeting a competent student with a visual impairment, the individual might not visualize this student in the "university potential" category, despite the student's demonstrated competence.

Prior to meeting a student with a visual impairment, each individual will have a category containing beliefs relevant to those who are visually impaired. Therefore, knowing a child has a visual impairment may often have a potent effect upon how an adult or a classmate perceives all aspects of this child's performance and behaviour. Allport (1958) described labels such as "visually impaired" as those of "primary potency."

> Some labels, such as "blind man," are exceedingly salient and powerful. They tend to prevent classification, or even cross-classification. These symbols act like shrieking sirens, deafening us to all finer discriminations that we might otherwise perceive. Each label we use, especially those of primary potency, distracts our attention from concrete reality. The living, breathing, complex individual—the ultimate unit of human nature—is lost to sight. The label magnifies one attribute out of all proportion to its true significance, and masks other important attributes of the individual. (p. 175-176)

Therefore, on one hand, there is a need to sort and categorize information about the world in order to organize one's thinking and subsequent behaviour. On the other hand, once the image or conception has emerged, it frequently remains relatively stable despite the introduction of new information. As a group or society, a shared image becomes the standard or stereotype for the way most group members think about that image. "Whether favourable or unfavourable, a stereotype is an exaggerated belief associated with a category. Its function is to justify (rationalize) our conduct in relation to that category" (Allport, 1958,p. 191). As adults, either educators or parents, there is a need to examine beliefs and expectations relevant to those with disabilities because there is a real danger that these fears, superstitions, and prejudices will be transmitted to both students with an impairment and their peers.

Although a visual impairment may be only one attribute of an individual, it may become the most prominent one — one that can become stigmatizing. A stigma is an undesirable differentness having negative connotations which may result in a feeling of shame and inferior status (Nixon, 1991). Stereotypes and stigmas may result in the development of attitudes which appear to have a pervasive effect on the integration of those with disabilities not only in our schools but into society, in general.

Monbeck (1975) argued that visual impairment conveys a social stigma which is often viewed as a symbol of physical, social, emotional, and economic inferiority. He believed that the negative nature of the beliefs which have formed today's stereotype of the blind ensure an adverse effect on the status of those with a visual impairment. Frequently they are perceived to be powerless and dependent upon the benevolence of society for their survival. MacCuspie (1991) concluded that even as early as elementary school, the label "visually impaired" can have a pervasive and negative effect upon the perceptions and meanings developed by classmates, educators and parents of visually impaired children. The negative influence of this label can be potent even in the face of evidence to the contrary, i.e., despite the high academic performance of the student with a visual impairment. The label, visually impaired, can obscure the perceptions and the meanings others create in relation to those with a visual impairment and contribute to lowered expectations for their social, physical and academic performance.

Despite the great heterogeneity inherent within the population of those with a visual impairment, they are generally considered as a singular group by society. Yet, unlike members of many other minorities (e.g., ethnic groups or religious affiliations), the individual who is blind does not have the benefit of close association with family members experiencing the day-to-day effects of their minority status (Monbeck, 1975). The student with a visual impairment in an integrated setting is unlikely to have a single peer with whom to share the experience of being visually impaired. Not only are those with a visual impairment apt to be judged on the basis of existing stereotypes, they are also often deprived of the support which is traditionally associated with affiliation with "one's own kind."

Although the treatment of the visually impaired in society has improved dramatically during the past century, beliefs about visual impairment and those with this condition unfortunately do not seem to have reflected a corresponding change. The dismal employment statistics for those with a visual impairment are but one indication of society's failure to integrate this minority. Therefore, as the principles of integration are implemented, the stereotypes and stigmas associated with visual impairment or blindness must be acknowledged. It is only then that a plan to address and change attitudes and beliefs detrimental to the positive acceptance of difference and social integration can be devised and implemented.

Social Relationships

By nature, humans are gregarious. From the initial bonding between parent and child, there is a strong, pervasive bias to form social relationships with others (Cairns, 1986). This tendency continues to evolve throughout all stages of life. Beginning in the preschool years, children's peers play an increasingly central role in the social world and social development of children. Early friendships based on proximity and shared play interests set the foundation for stable, complex relationships characteristic of the personal and professional lives of adults.

Social development and the skills essential to appropriate social interaction reflect a level of variability similar to that within other aspects of human development. Social development must be viewed as a dynamic process changing in response to life-long changes in body chemistry, cognitive development and experiences with social interactions in thousands of situations. Gender, age, personality, cultural expectations, and numerous other factors have been shown to influence social development and the types of relationships that evolve. Regardless of the obvious complexity of social development, positive social interactions and acceptance or inclusion by one's peers are essential components for the healthy social-emotional or affective development of us all.

Social Acceptance Versus Tolerance

Those who have advocated and advanced the integration of students with disabilities never intended for these children to be deprived of the joys and sorrows of friendship. Yet, the majority of researchers examining the social acceptance of students with disabilities in integrated settings have reported tolerance of these individuals by their peers rather than inclusive or accepting relationships (Gresham, 1982; MacCuspie, 1991; Quintal, 1986). Tolerance is characterized by indifference to or ignoring of one's presence; whereas acceptance, for the purposes of this book, refers to a relationship between a child and her/his peer group which is characterized by active and spontaneous interaction. Acceptance is reflected in the perception by the group that the child is an appropriate playmate or workmate, one who should be routinely included in classroom and playground activities. An accepted child is infrequently discouraged from participating in the typical group events of the school day.

Inherent in the concept of normalization is the belief that individuals with an impairment will have opportunities for meaningful participation in the everyday world of the culture in which they reside. For school age children with disabilities, integration into the typical activities of public school placements necessitates integration into the social world of their peers who are not disabled. Integration without social acceptance and the development of positive relationships with peers condemns children to loneliness and robs them of the joys of childhood—experiences which can never be recaptured.

An essential component of integration is the positive acceptance of difference which is demonstrated when a student with a disability becomes a meaningful and contributing member of the class. As Johnson and Johnson (1980) contended:

> *Experience with a broad range of peers is not a superficial luxury to be enjoyed by some students and not by others, but rather an absolute necessity for maximal achievement and healthy cognitive and social development. Social interactions with peers may be the*

primary relationships within which development and socialization take place. (p. 90)

Schools are the principal environment for students to develop effective social skills and experience positive social relationships because they are the main source of social interaction with peers available to most children. Schools are social organizations which function as a primary socializing agent for youth during their formative years. Upon entering school, children must learn a new set of rules relevant to the roles and role relationships in a given classroom (Hargreaves, 1975). From a social-psychological perspective, schools provide children the opportunity to learn and practice new roles, ones which slowly evolve into those adult roles they will eventually assume in society.

For children, social acceptance is essential to the development of a healthy self-concept. The social environment is of fundamental importance in the development of the sense of self. A student's developing self-concept is influenced by the position occupied in the classroom and the status associated with this position (Tuttle, 1984). Consequently, the peer group has a significant role to play in the socialization process of each member of a class (Davies, 1982; Pollard, 1985). The desire to belong is a basic and powerful attribute which will be reflected in the dynamic learning process inherent to the development of a sense of self. Because one's self-concept is derived, in part, from one's perception of how others view her/him, this will influence, in turn, one's behaviour toward others (Tuttle, 1984). High self-esteem is a consequence of being openly valued and accepted by others. In an integrated setting, if peer relationships are to be a constructive influence, "they must promote feelings of belonging, acceptance, support, and caring, as opposed to feelings of rejection, abandonment, and alienation" (Johnson & Johnson, 1984, p. 91).

As parents and educators, the importance of having expectations that children with disabilities will have meaningful, social relationships is significant. Beliefs held by adults will underpin and guide their behaviour. It is their action or inaction which will determine whether or not students with disabilities will experience social acceptance by their peers. As readers consolidate the concepts and issues discussed in this chapter, the complexities associated with integration may seem to be overwhelming. Yet, examples of successful integration exist in our schools. The decisive factor is that "success comes from doing—not from hoping."

2

Social Development - A General Overview

Introduction

Perhaps no area of human development reflects such diversity as does social behaviour. Given that, it seems ironic that the pressure to be the same as one's peers appears to be such a powerful force throughout most of our lives. During the life-long process of personality and social development, we respond to what seems to be a natural instinct to interact with others. As mentioned previously in Chapter 1, there is a strong, pervasive bias to form social relationships and interact with others regardless of our stage of development —infant, toddler, teenager, or senior citizen. Since it is primarily during the school years that children learn the social skills and behaviours which prepare them for adulthood, it is critical that teachers and parents understand the importance of and learn how to monitor and enhance the social development, interaction and peer acceptance of children.

There are many aspects of social development, e.g., self-concept, self-esteem, personality, temperament, prosocial behaviour, anti-social behaviour, social cognition, morality, and empathy. These aspects of our being are not autonomous nor are they stable across time and context; rather, social development and behaviour is variable, responding in sometimes unpredictable ways to a multiplicity of factors such as heredity, cultural norms, and social context. Indeed, human difference is what makes our fellow beings so intriguing. It is through the process of interaction with others that the social being evolves.

Social Interaction

When a child is born, the first act of social interaction is known as bonding. Typically, this is a shared experience between parent and child which sets the stage for an intimate, long-term relationship known as attachment. This positive, affective bond develops seemingly automatically as parent and child interact shortly after the child's birth and during the early months of their new life together. Ainsworth (1982) proposes four phases of the attachment process. Phase 1, *initial preattachment*, is characterized by the child's "proximity-promoting" behaviours such as crying, smiling, and staring at the adult's face. This behaviour is intended to attract or maintain the adult's attention and is elicited indiscriminately to all caregivers in the child's environment. *Attachment in the making*, phase 2 of the process, occurs around 3 months of age when the child can be seen to respond more enthusiastically to those who are familiar than to a new face. In phase 3, at about 6 to 7 months of age, the child enters into a *clear-cut attachment*. One person, most often the primary caregiver, becomes the main recipient of the child's attention and is now actively sought out by the child. During this phase the child will use the person to whom they have become attached as a "safe base" when they are threatened. In an unfamiliar situation or when a stranger enters the scene, the child will look to the face of the preferred person to obtain clues relevant to the nature of the situation. This action is known as social referencing. Typical of this phase is the child's display of fear of strangers and objections to being separated from the person to whom they are attached.

Phase 4 is the *multiple attachment* stage when children begin to expand their range of attachments to other family members and those who frequent their world and interact with them. Usually by school age, parental attachment becomes less intense and the child's interest turns to social interaction with peers. As the child grows through adolescence, the attachment to parents may remain strong but the focus of the relationship is usually toward nurturing rather than the intimacy which comes to be characteristic of peer relationships. Within the context of these peer relationships, children practice, experiment with, and refine the social skills and understanding which contribute to a healthy adjustment during adult years.

Developmental Patterns of Social Interactions Among Children

The social behaviour of children generally follows somewhat predictable patterns or stages. Parents may be painfully aware, for example, of the rebellious behaviours associated with "the terrible twos" or the early teenage years. It is recognized that there is tremendous variability, growth, and change throughout any given period of social development. However, for the purposes of this text, social behaviour will be examined during the preschool, elementary, and secondary school (i.e., junior/senior high) years. As early as 6 months of age, children appear to express an interest in other infants. By a year and a half, children will play together with toys for short periods of time but prefer to play side by side rather than be involved in cooperative play. At approximately 3 or 4 years of age, when consistent play behaviour involving purposeful interaction with other children starts to emerge, the beginnings of friendships or selection of preferred playmates can be observed in about 50 percent of children (Bee, 1989). In general, however, early friendships appear to be based more on proximity and common interests in comparison to the more intimate friendships of older children. These later friendships are characterized by sharing of feelings, self-disclosure, trust, and loyalty. During the first few years of schooling, children appear to play with a number of different children. Individual, stable friendships usually begin to emerge during the second or third year of school as the children begin to focus more on the importance of peer interactions than child-adult relationships. The importance of acceptance by peers and being someone's "best friend" is of critical significance to children by the middle elementary school years (Berndt, 1983; MacCuspie, 1991). Although boys and girls may be seen playing together on the playground, for the most part elementary school friendships are highly sex-segregated. As well, boys tend to interact with groups of friends while girls, particularly toward later elementary years, develop more intimate, exclusive relationships.

Interactions of Junior and Senior High Youth

The junior high years are perhaps the most intense years in relation to the child's desire to belong to the peer group (Berndt, 1982). They are marked by a significant increase in the amount of time peers spend with one another either physically together or talking on the telephone. This stage of children's development is also frequently the period marked by the most intense conflict with parents as youth struggle with their emerging sense of independence (Bee, 1989). Because friendship is an egalitarian relationship, that is, participants perceive one another as equals, this relationship provides an opportunity to engage in the types of social interactions characteristic of egalitarianism. These interactions with peers, i.e., their equals, are in sharp contrast to hierarchical relationships, such as those between parent and child or teacher and student. Thus, egalitarian relationships provide the opportunity to experience and experiment with new aspects of interpersonal communication.

Researchers examining the way in which friendships evolve have reported that there appears to be a similarity of attributes and behaviours among those who are friends in early adolescence (Berndt, 1982). Attitude toward school, achievement level in school, and educational aspirations are attributes which tend to be shared by friends. Since adolescence is also the period in which many youth begin to experiment with drugs, alcohol, sexual relationships, and antisocial group behaviour, these interests also serve as opportunities to develop friendships. From a behaviourial perspective, it appears friends tend to share similar orientations toward the prevalent adolescent culture in terms of dress, music, educational, and recreational pursuits.

The influence of the peer group on behaviour and perceptions, very strong throughout the entire years of schooling, seems to peak during the junior high years. Although adolescents have stable, individual friendships during this period, they often spend time together in groups of four to six individuals which researchers refer to as cliques (Bee, 1989). These are same-sex groups characterized by a strong cohesiveness and an intimate sharing of thoughts and feelings. As boy-girl relationships become more prevalent, heterosexual cliques and loose associations of couples become more common for high school students. Throughout adolescence, individual friendships are typically stable and intimate. These relationships give teenagers a "safe base" similar in some ways to that provided by parents during the child's preschool years.

Positive and Negative Interactions Among Children

Children who have secure attachments with their parents seem to be skillful in establishing relationships with their peers (Asher, Renshaw & Hymel, 1982). As children begin to spend increasingly greater amounts of time interacting with peers than with adults, acceptance by the group becomes increasingly important and requires the addition and cultivation of new social skills and concepts. Hartup (1984) contended that rejection by one's peers during the elementary school years is highly correlated with behaviour and/or emotional problems in both the teenage and adult years.

Researchers have identified a number of factors associated with popularity among elementary school children. Examples of such factors include behaviour which is friendly, supportive, outgoing and not aggressive or disruptive; a physically attractive appearance; and success in games, sports and academic achievement (Bee, 1989). However, the crucial element in popularity during the elementary years is how a child behaves toward peers. Children who are gregarious, not critical, and who display an interest in their peers are observed to be those sought out by others (Bee, 1989). As children reach adolescence, popularity continues to be associated with those perceived to be most intelligent, dominant, and attractive. But, as in the elementary years, popularity is most strongly associated with individuals who demonstrate positive and supportive behaviour toward others.

Social Cognition

Simply defined, social cognition is the understanding of social relationships. Theorists from the cognitive perspective believe children's social competence is a reflection of their level of cognitive or intellectual development. They contend that social skills such as perspective-taking (i.e., the ability to comprehend the feelings and circumstances of others) are developmental and emerge in conjunction with increased cognitive understanding. Researchers (Berndt, 1982; Kurdek & Krile, 1982) have found that children with average and above average scores on tests measuring understanding of individuals and the concept of friendship were more apt to be involved in mutual friendships than were those with lower scores. Bee (1989) stated that there appears to be a correlation between social cognition and behaviour. Teenagers who scored well on tests of social cognition (e.g., those measuring empathy, friendship analysis, and moral reasoning) were more likely to demonstrate moral or empathetic behaviour and were perceived to have positive friendships with peers.

Yet, social cognition must be distinguished from other facets of cognition because it involves interaction with other humans who may act in unpredictable ways (Bee, 1989). For example, individuals frequently do not disclose their true feelings or may respond according to learned social rules or roles. Learning to interpret nonverbal communication which is contrary to the verbal message being sent (e.g., a facial expression indicating anguish), or learning to identify vocally expressed emotions such as disappointment or enthusiasm are aspects of social cognition which develop through routine interaction in a variety of relationships such as friendships, child-parent discussions, and conflicts with others. Therefore, the quantity and variety of social interaction experienced by children can be of crucial importance in the development of social competence.

This is not to suggest that children must reach a specific level of social understanding to participate in meaningful, positive social relationships. The mutual pleasure experienced in the play between an infant and an older sibling would certainly contradict this. However, it does alert one to the probability that aspects of children's relationships, such as friendships, are developmental and will change with learning, maturity, and experience.

The recent emphasis on social cognition as it relates to the social behaviour of children is of critical importance to the planning of programs to assist children who are not well accepted by their peer group. Not only must educators address the social understanding of the "at risk" child but also ensure the child's peers understand the potential interpretation problems being experienced by the unpopular child. The classroom must provide a safe environment for children to observe and learn social skills under the direction and guidance of their teachers and more proficient peers. That is, affective as well as cognitive development must become a classroom goal.

Pupil Culture and Its Implications for Social Integration

The integration of children with disabilities into regular public school classrooms has been a phenomena which has become increasingly promoted during the past few decades (Winzer, Rogow, & David, 1987). Proposed to be both a positive movement to enhance the opportunity for these children to experience and learn from "normal" role models and to encourage students who are not disabled to become more compassionate and tolerant of individual difference, integration has been endorsed by its advocates as the experience which will ensure appropriate educational opportunities for those with disabilities. However, as educators have experienced integration of the disabled and as researchers have documented results, it has become increasingly evident that the physical proximity of those with disabilities and their regular classroom peers does not necessarily result in social integration (Gresham, 1982; Hoben & Lindstom, 1980; Quintal, 1986).

There is a consensus among teachers of the visually impaired and parents of these students that many of these children experience limited social integration in the regular classroom (MacCuspie, 1992; Sacks & Reardon, 1989). Much of the research addressing the social adaptation of those who have a visual impairment has been focused on the deficits identified as characteristic of this group (e.g., limited access to nonverbal cues, mannerisms). The structuring aspects of the social environment, the complexities of social interaction, the interactive nature of interpersonal relationships, and the impact of society's treatment of those who are visually impaired as an inferior minority are only implicit in some of this research.

As members of a regular public school classroom, children who are visually impaired are immersed in a culture which is exclusive to children, that is, pupil culture. This is the culture to which they must be socialized if acceptance by peers and associated benefits (e.g., friendships, acceptance to peer groups) are to result.

Schooling literature would suggest that pupil culture, most evident on the playground or outside the classroom, has several significant functions relevant to the social development and interaction of students (Davies, 1982; Pollard, 1985; Woods, 1979). First, pupil culture develops as a defensive resource for pupils against teachers and other adults. Children live in a world which is both directed and dominated by adults. Pollard (1985, p. 49) suggested that within the camaraderie of pupil culture, children are provided a "source of support, security, and positive esteem which is to a great extent insulated from the often threatening experience of teacher-dominated classroom processes or of parental strictures."

A second function of pupil culture is to address problems of internal integration such as group boundaries, that is, who belongs and who does not. The initial development of groups can be observed as early as the middle elementary years. By junior high school, groups associated around such interests as sports, high or low academic achievement, music, or other recreational pursuits are evident. Depending upon the geographic location and the particular generation, groups are variously labelled within pupil culture by such names as "jocks", "dweebs", "geeks", and "preppies". By senior high school such groups are well defined and highly exclusive to outsiders.

A third function of pupil culture, closely associated with the establishment of group boundaries, is that associated with the benefits of group membership. Insiders or those who belong to the group receive special treatment and develop a sense of identity —they are an accepted and recognized member of the group. Those who belong to the group need not seek out others with whom to interact since group members are usually readily available and tend to share common interests with one another. Fellow members provide a "safe base" and a reliable source of friends. Those who do not belong to the group, often known as "outsiders", do not have access to such friendship cliques. Frequently those viewed to be outside the group are rejected, neglected, or even treated with hostility by group members. On elementary playgrounds, in particular, students who are rebuffed by their peers face an additional consequence of their rejection. They are often emotionally or physically abused by other children who are hoping to improve their own popularity by prominent demonstrations of dislike for rejected children, that is, those outside established friendship circles (MacCuspie, 1991).

The fourth function of pupil culture is to provide an arena for children to legitimize their perception of the world. Here, the commonsense knowledge of childhood, shared values, and perceptions will be generated (Pollard, 1985). Children frequently generate their own explanations to resolve the contradictions and dilemmas which infringe on their world. For example, during a recent visit to an elementary school, a pair of grade two children were overheard discussing the method used in their school to assign children to the classrooms of specific teachers. These two children had decided that since, in their experience, they were assigned to a "nice" teacher's class every second year that this was how placement decisions were made. The conversation included future predictions of the character of the teacher to whom they would be assigned in each of the remaining four years of their elementary school education. For these two students, their perceptions were a shared reality at this point in their development. They genuinely believed that adults organized class placement following this pattern. Davies (1982) contended that the culture of childhood is a reflection of the distinct manner in which children interpret the world, not an immature adult version, but rather one which is embedded in the different ways children perceive and experience their world.

A fifth function of pupil culture is to generate collective strategies which will help children to cope with the adult-directed world (Pollard, 1985). The following story, written by a grade one student, provides an example of a common strategy children develop to cope with the dominating world of adults:

The Talking Hotdog

> It was Friday, hotdog day for the Grade 1 class. *"Hotdogs,"* called Mrs. Smith, their teacher. When Katie got her hotdog, someone said, *"Please don't eat me!"*
> *"Who said that?"* said Katie
> *"I did,"* said the hotdog.
> *"Wow!"* said Katie. *"I didn't know hotdogs could talk. What is your name?"*
> *"Melanie,"* said the hotdog.
> *"Can all the hotdogs talk?"* asked Katie.
> *"No, certainly not,"* said the hotdog.
> *"Then, how...,"* Katie started but the hotdog interrupted.
> *"I got sprinkled by magic,"* Melanie said.
> Katie said, *"Can I tell Megan?"* *"Yes,"* said the hotdog. *"Certainly, yes. But don't tell grownups."*

Then Katie felt a tap on the shoulder. Then she woke up. *"It was only a dream,"* said Katie.
The End

The information which can and cannot be shared with teachers and parents, i.e., "grownups", is well known among children, as is the consequence of breaking this rule and telling an adult. Children who appear to have difficulty learning the sometimes subtle rules of pupil culture are often those who appear to be less accepted by their peers.

Following extensive studies of social relationships within junior and senior high schools, Woods (1983) outlined three frequently occurring themes inherent to pupil or childhood culture—competence, relationships (i.e., friendships), and status. Competence refers to the child's ability to see herself/himself in relation to peers and to act according to their expectations. A socially competent child is able to understand her/his social identity in relation to peers and to acquire the skills necessary for the successful or appropriate interaction within multiple social situations encountered during a typical day, such as waiting at the bus stop with other students; initiating the substitute teacher to the rules of the classroom; participating in lunch hour activities or a Friday night party at a friend's house. In order to become competent, a flexible repertoire of behaviours appropriated with various roles must be learned by students (Sieber, 1979a). For example, a child must understand the discretion and secrecy to be used when classroom interaction is not permitted by the teacher, the procedure to follow when joining existing groups of interacting students, the behaviours to use to initiate play or to joke with a classmate, and the change in demeanour required when associating with members of the opposite gender. To interact successfully within pupil culture, students need to know the status items of the pupil culture, that is, what is or is not important or meaningful. Thus, social competence within the pupil culture requires the child to learn both the negotiated rules of conduct for behaviour within the group and the value placed on various aspects of the culture.

Friendships and Their Functional Qualities

The nature of friendships vary from those characteristic of the early elementary school years which are based more on physical accessibility to those of teenagers which tend to focus on psychological compatibility, trust, and loyalty. Despite this variation, the functional qualities of friendship are relatively stable. First, friendship provides a source of companionship. When you have a friend you have someone to interact with during recess, to be your partner when the teachers wants students to work in pairs, and to play or interact with after school. One of the most dreaded childhood experiences is to be alone on the playground or to be standing alone in the corridor amidst other children who are laughing, playing, and seemingly having fun.

A second functional quality of friendship is its capacity to provide a source of stimulation. Teachers are acutely aware of the amount of information which is shared among classmates. Children acquire information about the travels and family experiences of their peers, television programs viewed and their content, books read and enjoyed, antics of older and younger siblings or other relatives, and other various extra-curricular activities. Many life-long interests and hobbies are initially introduced through interaction with one's peers. Beyond this rather informal source of stimulation is the role social interaction plays in cognitive, social, physical, and linguistic development. Children who are routinely left alone on the sidelines are, through exclusion from the activities of others, missing an extraordinary amount of time practising and refining the skills of social interaction and effective communication, motor co-ordination and physical fitness, and intellectual processing and problem solving. In short, we learn through interaction with our environment and the amount of time we are effectively interacting with this environment will have a significant effect upon the amount of learning and maturation that occurs.

Physical support is a third functional quality of friendship. Friends help when one is threatened by a bully on the playground, being taunted by peers in the corridor, or afraid to walk alone at night. Some activities (e.g., tennis, building a tree house) require the physical presence of a companion while others (e.g., biking, camping) are just more fun or safer in the company of a friend. How often do we decide against participating in an activity because we have "no one to go with?" This physical and emotional support provided by friends is frequently essential to our willingness to try unfamiliar activities or to meet new challenges.

Another important functional quality of friendship is that of ego support. Friends are an invaluable source of positive reinforcement in the form of praise and encouragement. Even when one makes an error or misjudgment, friends are much less harsh in their criticism or negative reactions than are those who are not considered to be friends (MacCuspie, 1991). Critical to the development of high self-esteem is the need to receive positive messages about our behaviour and our value from others (Tuttle, 1984). Thus, for children and youth, peers are a major source of positive reinforcement and encouragement and have a critical influence upon the development of self-esteem.

Closely associated with the ego support provided by friendship is the functional quality of social comparison. Humans seem to have a pervasive tendency to compare appearance, behaviour, and performance with that of their peers. Friendship provides a safe environment in which to make comparisons and receive feedback. We can compete with friends without expecting to experience harsh consequences when we don't "measure up." As well, friends provide advice and encouragement relevant to how we compare with others and ways to improve our status.

The sixth and final functional quality of friendship to be considered is that of intimacy and affection. Friendship has been conceptualized as an "affective bond, a relationship charged with positive feelings" (Fine, 1981, p. 41). If parental love is viewed as a necessity for healthy emotional development, then friendship must also be considered an essential experience for school-age children as they spend increasingly less time under the direct influence of parents. As children struggle to become independent of parents they need an alternate source of support, that is, peers. Mutual affection in a relationship is both a pleasurable and beneficial experience. Why do children want so badly to be part of a group and to have friends? Because it's a wonderful feeling to be accepted and valued by others. The following excerpt is from a radio interview with a ten year old, congenitally blind, grade five student. It demonstrates the intensity of the longing to have a friend.

> *When I grow up I think I'll either have a seeing eye dog or use a cane. But, I think a seeing eye dog is best because, you know, it's a friend and someone who can help you at the same time.*
>
> *Some of my friends, well, I have one friend and she tells jokes...One of my friends used to lie to me just because I was blind and I didn't think that was fair. I mean, just because I'm blind doesn't mean people have to play little tricks on me. Blind people, visually impaired people, should be treated just like normal people. Just because they're blind doesn't mean they can't do anything different from normal people. We're just the same only we can't see.*
>
> *I usually don't notice but my fifth sense tells me. Because I realize what they're doing later. Like, he said there was a bees' nest on a little log on my steps and there wasn't. I mean, he played these silly little tricks on me just because I was blind. It made me feel angry because, I mean, if I could have a true friend, a best friend that wouldn't lie to me, I think I'd be happy. I'd probably be the happiest visually impaired person in the world.*

Friendship is a natural component of pupil culture. Although friendships influence the quantity and quality of the extra-curricular activities of a child from a very early age, it is important to recognize the role friendships play in the classroom as well. In classrooms where the teacher must respond to the needs of twenty-five to thirty-five children, it is frequently difficult for teachers to provide the assistance needed in a timely manner. A child who has friends can usually obtain assistance from another child but the child who is rejected by peers will not necessarily be offered the same support. Thus, in the classroom a child who does not have friends is potentially at risk both in terms of social and cognitive development. The main functional qualities of friendship may vary in intensity between class and extra-curricular life but are, none-the-less, critical to the healthy social development of students in either situation.

Status

Status is the third theme inherent to pupil culture identified by Woods (1983). Pollard (1985) suggested that the type of identity which a child creates and which then becomes associated with that child by peers results in a particular status within the group. The level of this status may be seen as the social outcome of friendship relations and social competence. Hargreaves (1975) outlined three dimensions of status within a group which contribute to one's position in the status hierarchy or system of valuing individuals within the group. First, sociometric status is concerned with the degree to which individuals are liked by or popular with other group members. The more popular students have a higher status in the group than do the unpopular children, hence, are more often sought out as friends. Second, social power or influence, concerned with the capacity of one individual to control the behaviour of another, affects one's status in the group. For example, a student with effective leadership qualities can have tremendous influence on who is included or excluded from activities as well as the status which is granted to the activities themselves. The third dimension of status is prestige and is related to specific positions within the formal group. The class president or the captain of the ball team is granted a degree of prestige that differs from that granted individuals holding positions of lesser esteem (e.g., secretary, bat boy). Holding a valued position in the school or class will increase the probability of developing positive social relationships with other interested students.

Within pupil culture, children develop a pecking order or status which tends to be relatively stable over time (Davies, 1982; Fine, 1981). This fact accentuates the importance of early intervention to prevent a child from being excluded by peers. Once a child has a reputation as being an unpopular classmate it is extremely difficult to change this perception among the other members of the group. In rural areas of our country where it is possible for students to be with the same peers throughout their entire twelve or thirteen years of schooling, a student who is identified as unpopular during the early elementary grades may live with an inescapable sentence (i.e., undesirable companion) for the duration of her/his school years.

Adults often make the horrendous mistake of underestimating the value and importance children place on friendship, as well as the critical function friendship plays in social and intellectual development. Frequently the significance of children's friendships are trivialized by viewing them as being erratic or immature relationships — different from those of adulthood. Parents and educators must begin to insist that the same importance granted to academic progress in our schools is given to the affective development of all children.

Social Acceptance/Integration of Children with Disabilities

The integration of students with disabilities into the regular classrooms of public schools is a basic principle of contemporary special education. The number of children with disabilities enrolled in public schools during the last two decades has dramatically increased. Those who have ardently promoted integration anticipated frequent, spontaneous interaction between children with disabilities and their classmates. Increased social acceptance by and exposure to students in the regular classroom was expected to increase the disabled child's imitation of appropriate behaviour. However, as these children have had the opportunity to both attend public schools and participate in regular classes, it has become increasingly evident that the physical proximity of disabled and nondisabled children does not necessarily result in these positive outcomes. In fact, unfortunately, social isolation rather than social integration more often appears to be the consequence of mainstreaming students with disabilities (Gresham, 1982; MacMillan & Morrison, 1984; Sabornie, 1985). The majority of studies examining the social acceptance and status of children with disabilities in integrated settings report that these students interact less frequently and more negatively with their peers who are not disabled and tend to be ignored or rejected by them (Gresham, 1982; Hoben, 1980; Quintal, 1986). Despite the inconclusiveness and sometimes contradictory findings of the research, it appears that social integration has not been the natural outcome of enrolling children with disabilities in regular classrooms. What is evident from an examination of the research is that educators must begin to look beyond the child as the source of problems in integrated settings and begin to look more closely at the nature of the social environment which has come to characterize schools.

Improving the Social Acceptance of Students with Disabilities

In special education classes, the most common approach to improving the social acceptance of students with disabilities has been to attempt to teach the student specific social skills, such as how to join a group or control aggressive behaviours. This process has been characterized by the identification of those social skills which were lacking or delayed, the selection of specific skills to be taught, some form of structured teaching to develop the skills, and the evaluation of mastery of the skill in the natural environment. For students with disruptive or aggressive behaviours, the programs have frequently focused on the elimination of specific undesirable behaviours, such as hitting or making derogatory comments.

In regular education classrooms, teachers have traditionally taught social skills which enhance classroom control, such as raising the hand before speaking or listening without interrupting the speaker. The emphasis has not necessarily been on teaching social skills which will improve a student's social competence in interaction with peers or which might be expected to generalize to situations outside the classroom but rather on those social behaviours which contribute to an orderly learning environment. Students with disruptive behaviour have been a major concern to regular classroom teachers since extra time and energy is required to deal with their behaviour; behaviour which usually interferes with the learning of both the disruptive student and her/his classmates. Students who are withdrawn, shy or neglected by their peers frequently have not received any formal assistance in addressing their social interaction difficulties because they do not usually impede the progress of the class. Teachers, although sympathetic, often feel a sense of helplessness in dealing with such children because they believe they do not have the training or qualifications to deal appropriately with the situation, the time available to provide the individual instruction required, or the support of administrators or parents in providing "non-academic" instruction.

As students with disabilities have become integrated into the regular classroom and educators and parents have become more aware of their social integration needs, there has been a growing pressure to address the social isolation which many of these students experience. A focus on social skills training, traditionally incorporated in programs for adolescents and adults with disabilities, is beginning to be promoted for all children at the preschool and elementary levels. Early intervention can prevent the development of inappropriate behaviour and structure experiences which will promote the growth of social competence. Researchers and educators have also become aware of the need to use strategies which ensure the student is able to generalize newly acquired social skills from the instructional situation to the natural environment both in the classroom and during extra-curricular activities. Those who once focused instruction on changing the behaviour of the student with the disability have now come to realize that the nature of the social environment and the behaviour of its participants (i.e., peers, teachers, principals, parents) have an essential role to play if real gains in social acceptance and interaction of students with disabilities are to be realized. It is now obvious to educators that social integration will not be achieved by merely teaching social skills to students with disabilities. If social skills instruction is to have a significant effect upon the long-term social behaviour or social acceptance of these students, the social environment in which interaction occurs must be analyzed and, in most cases, modified.

In conclusion, integration for school-age children with disabilities necessitates social integration into the social world of their peers who are not disabled. This is the social environment educators must examine and modify if social acceptance by peers is to be a benefit of integration enjoyed by students with impairments. If society is to realize the benefits of an inclusive school system, it must take the opportunity integration presents to improve the learning environment for all students. Research indicates that there are few classrooms where there is not at least one rejected or neglected child (MacCuspie, 1991; Nezer, Nezer & Siperstein, 1985). The plight of these children is evidence that educators need to address the affective as well as the cognitive and physical development of their students. That the integration of students with disabilities could provide the catalyst to modify the mainstream so as to enhance a positive learning environment for all students, is an optimistic note upon which to begin our exploration of the social acceptance and interaction of students with a visual impairment in an integrated school setting.

3

Implications of Visual Impairment for Social Interaction

Introduction

The child with a visual impairment is, first of all, a child. Visual impairment is but one attribute of this individual, therefore, many things are shared in common with other children. Like all children, the child with a visual impairment will have specific learning strengths and weaknesses, individual interests and needs, and particular likes and dislikes. The child with a visual impairment may be happy-go-lucky or serious, passive or active, chubby or thin. Of one thing to be certain, the child with a visual impairment will have the same need for emotional support, intellectual stimulation, and physical activity as other children.

In addition to these typical childhood attributes and needs, a child with a visual impairment will have some unique needs associated with the limitations a reduction or loss of vision creates in relation to development and learning. With appropriate and timely intervention many of the negative influences can be compensated or overcome. However, in some aspects of development, children with a visual impairment will experience and interact with their environment in very different ways than will those who are fully sighted. An understanding of the potential differences in development and of the implications these differences may have is a prerequisite for those striving to enhance the social interaction and acceptance of children who are visually impaired.

The Visually Impaired Population

Visual impairment is a condition commonly associated with the elderly because of the number of visual disorders related to the aging process (e.g., cataracts, macular degeneration). Indeed, a majority of the population who are visually impaired is comprised of adults over fifty years of age.

In both Canada and the United States, the number of children with a visual impairment who are of school age is estimated to be approximately 0.14 percent or 14 per 10,000 school children. The incidence of total blindness is 0.01 percent or 1 per 10,000. Visual impairment is considered to be a low-incidence condition in comparison to the incidence of other types of exceptionalities such as intellectual impairments or learning disabilities. For the purposes of this text, one is considered to have a visual impairment if corrected visual acuity is less than 20/70 in the better eye or restrictions in peripheral vision resulting in a field of 20 degrees or less are present, regardless of visual acuity. In this book, those who are totally blind are included in the term visual impairment.

With respect to intellectual functioning, the visually impaired as a group exhibit a wide range of abilities. Within this population there is a broad range from those who are gifted to those who have profound, multiple impairments (Scholl, 1986). As medical technology has improved, the number of children with severe, multiple disabilities who survive the early critical years has increased dramatically. Since visual impairment is frequently one of several disabilities experienced by this group, this has changed the composition of the visually impaired population as it was known several decades ago (Winzer, 1990). The extreme heterogeneity which characterizes the population with a visual impairment within North America today may well contribute to greater misconceptions among the public than has been the case in the past.

The Optical System and Visual Impairment

The optical system is comprised of the eye, the optical pathway and the brain. Visual impairment may result when there is damage to any part of the optical system. Injury, disease, or malformation of any part of the eyeball can cause varying degrees of vision loss or total blindness. The optic nerve leading from the eye to the brain can be the source of damage resulting in vision loss. When vision loss is a result of damage to the visual cortex, the area of the brain where visual messages are interpreted, the condition is known as cortical visual impairment. Because of the complexity of the optical system, there are many different types of visual impairment and associated functional implications. For example, a visual impairment involving a significant loss in peripheral vision (i.e., the field of vision) but good remaining visual acuity (i.e., central vision) will have a profound effect upon the ease with which one can move throughout the environment but may not seriously detract from the ability to read regular size print.

The measure of either visual acuity or peripheral vision, however, gives little indication of how a specific individual with a visual impairment will function. Just as children without a visual impairment learn to interpret the world through sensory input and from a variety of experiences, a child with a visual impairment learns to use the visual information received in conjunction with other sensory cues (e.g., auditory, tactile) to process information from the environment. Visual efficiency is a term used to describe a person's degree of skill in using vision to access information from the environment. Two individuals with the same eye condition and visual loss may function very differently because of the level of visual efficiency each has developed.

Corn (1985) outlined three dimensions of visual functioning which influence the level of visual efficiency an individual may achieve. First, visual abilities such as acuity, peripheral vision, and colour perception will determine the amount of visual information one receives. Second, individual attributes of a given person such as intellectual ability, perception, and psychological make-up (e.g., motivation) will influence how this individual interprets and processes the information. Third, environmental cues such as colour, contrast, and illumination will effect the quantity and quality of information received. All these aspects of the individual and the environment interact to create the level of visual efficiency, hence visual functioning attained. For example, a child who has been exposed to a variety of preschool experiences and expected to explore the environment and be relatively independent will, in all probability, demonstrate much better visual functioning than a child with a similar visual impairment who has been overprotected and discouraged from independent exploration and interaction with the environment.

Factors Influencing Social Interaction of Children With a Visual Impairment

Findings of much of the research focusing on those who are visually impaired tend to be vague, inconclusive, and contradictory (Warren, 1984). Two major factors are generally believed to be related to this problem. First, the majority of research on visual impairment has been undertaken using the scientific methods associated with statistical analysis, strict sampling procedures, and an emphasis on objectivity. The nature of visual impairment creates major difficulties from this research perspective. As the prevalence of visual impairment in the school-age population is so low, getting access to random samples or matching on specific variables (e.g., visual acuity, visual efficiency, IQ, achievement) is an onerous undertaking. Consequently, attempting to establish norms relevant to the school-age population with a visual impairment is extremely difficult. Compounding these problems is the absence of a standard definition of visual impairment for use in research. Legal blindness includes a range from total vision loss to varying degrees of functional or partial vision. Many studies include children with visual acuities below 20/70 but better than 20/200. These research subjects are not considered within the realm of legal blindness, i.e., having a visual acuity of less than 20/200, but they may often qualify for special education services because they experience difficulties similar to those who are more severely visually impaired.

The second factor contributing to the reliability of research involving those with a visual impairment is the extreme heterogeneity of the school-age population who are visually impaired. Variables such as the severity of loss, total or partial; the age of onset, congenital or adventitious; the nature of onset, gradual or sudden; intelligence and social adjustment; and the presence of associated physical or sensory impairments, all contribute to the extreme heterogeneity of this population and, for researchers, significant problems with reliability and generalization of findings.

Despite the inconclusive or vague findings characteristic of much of the research involving those who are visually impaired, both researchers and professionals have consistently identified a number of considerations which are important when examining the social development, interaction and learning of children who are visually impaired. These include the effects or implications associated with the limited or lack of access to visual information on the following:

- early parent-child relationships
- acquisition of social knowledge
- learning and using visual cues
- feedback through nonverbal communication
- physical development and agility
- cultural norms associated with communication patterns
- practice and refinement of interpersonal skills.

Also to be considered are those factors inherent to the interaction of an individual who is visuallly impaired in a society created by and for those who are fully sighted. They are as follows:

- perceptions associated with mannerisms or stereotypic behaviours (e.g., rocking, eye pressing)
- distinct facial features or appearance
- negative attitudes toward those with disabilities
- interaction stress
- contextual factors such as the degree of teacher acceptance or the method of instruction.

These twelve considerations, although inextricably interrelated in the social environment of the classroom, will be discussed individually to provide further clarification.

Early Parent-Child Relationships

In examining the early parent-child relationships of children with a severe visual impairment, it is necessary to look at both the emotional and the cognitive aspects of this relationship. The first act of social interaction is bonding. Over the first year it is expected that the child will develop attachments which are believed to contribute to future social adjustment and competence of the child. The birth of a child with a severe visual impairment is an extremely devastating time for parents. They must deal simultaneously with feelings of guilt, blame, anger, and denial and those of grief associated with the perceived loss of a "normal" child. As Nixon (1991) so aptly stated,

> *The ideas parents learned about impairments and impaired people before their experience with their impaired children do not suddenly become transformed by the discovery of impairment in their own families. Indeed ... negative stereotypes of the stigma of impairment help create the nightmare that follows the news that a child is impaired. (p. 16)*

The first few months following the birth of any child are typically characterized by a period of adjustment and stress. When a child has an impairment, parents can be overwhelmed by such things as the medical needs of the child, the reactions from family and friends, and the feelings of self-doubt concerning their ability to raise a child with an impairment. There is ample research to substantiate the potential negative effect visual impairment can have on early parent-child attachments (Fraiberg, 1977; Nixon, 1991). The initial time of bonding shortly after birth is often lost when the child is medically fragile and must be placed in intensive care or when the child is blind and does not respond visually to the mother's face. Visual impairment also interferes with the parent's ability to establish a method of nonverbal communication with the child. The child's inability to respond to facial expressions of the parent frequently leaves the parent feeling rejected by the child. Lack of a positive response, sends a negative message to parents convincing them that the child prefers to be left alone. Therefore, despite the best of intentions, a cycle of misinterpretation and miscommunication may begin and, unfortunately may become well established before the parents have received any assistance in understanding and dealing with the implications of vision loss on early attachments.

By examining Ainsworth's four phases of early attachment described in Chapter 2, the potential risks for a child with a visual impairment can be anticipated at each phase. For example, consider Phase 1, "initial preattachment", characterized by the child's "proximity-promoting" behaviours such as crying, smiling, and staring at the adult's face. The child with a visual impairment may cry when suddenly picked up or become startled when picked up in the middle of a crying bout because she did not hear the approaching caregiver. Children who are fully sighted smile instinctively in response to the visual configuration of the human face, however, when a child's acuity is reduced such that this configuration is indistinct or when a child receives no visual input, the natural stimulus for smiling behaviour is absent. Staring at the adult's face is obviously a behaviour which is unlikely to occur in a child with a severe visual impairment. Similarly, in phase 2, "attachment in the making", a child who is blind will not respond more enthusiastically to a familiar face than to a stranger's face. A child without a visual impairment would be expected to display excitement at seeing a familiar face. The expression of such excitement is not only gratifying for new parents but also reinforces the initiation of future parent-child interactions.

At Phase 3, "clear-cut attachment", one person becomes the primary recipient of the child's attention and is now actively sought out by the child, used as a "safe base" when threatened, and used to visually check out the person's reaction to new or unfamiliar situations. The child with a visual impairment may encounter tremendous difficulty in both physically locating and receiving messages from the person with whom they have made their primary attachment because the ability to locate the source of auditory cues develops much later than visual recognition skills (Fraiberg, 1977). The absence of a "safe base" for a child with a visual impairment discourages the active exploration of the environment essential to both physical and cognitive development and may result in the child being reluctant to move beyond a familiar area at any given time. Unless the caregiver becomes adept at providing verbal messages to the child who is facing an unfamiliar situation, the child with a visual impairment has little source of information upon which to base responses. Furthermore, because a 6 to 8 month old child has limited understanding of language, auditory cues cannot always compensate for the loss of nonverbal information the child who is fully sighted receives from the caregivers' expressions and responses.

During phase 4, the multiple attachment stage, children without disabilities usually begin to expand their attachments to family members and frequent visitors. The child who lacks the visual stimulation which motivates exploration of the environment is also apt to show disinterest in the people in this environment. These people must initiate the contact and invent strategies which invite the child to explore and interact. With the appropriate intervention and a parent physically and emotionally able to cope with the multitude of challenges to be faced during these early years, many of the negative effects of vision loss on early attachment can be prevented or reduced. Herein lies a significant dilemma. Much of the intervention provided by parents to stimulate the child's development requires them to act as a mediator between the child and her/his environment. By comparison, a child who is sighted learns many things incidentally through observation and imitation. For the child who is blind, a mediator must present objects, describe their characteristics and uses, and sometimes guide the child's hands as the objects are explored. Such intervention entails significantly more interaction with the child who is blind than is typically provided to children without such an impairment. Children may become very dependent upon the feedback parents provide, although this feedback has positive effects upon their learning and development. Yet, when this intervention does not take place and children with visual impairments experience ineffective interactions during the preschool years, they may develop inappropriate social behaviours which interfere with their opportunity to engage in social interaction typical of peers. Fraiberg (1977) has suggested that without intervention parents are unlikely to be able to provide the social environment which will allow the child to develop the basic trust or autonomy necessary to move to more advanced social development. Thus, it seems, even with intervention, children with visual impairments encounter different social experiences which may influence their development in unique ways.

Behaviours such as self-centredness, unresponsiveness to the concerns and interests of others, unusual language patterns, and preference for interaction with adults are frequently reported as negative social behaviours in children who are visually impaired (Sacks, Kekelis & Gaylord-Ross, 1992). Unfortunately, children with a visual impairment may enter school with these social behaviours which effectively isolate them from peers very early in their school careers and, without intervention, will continue to discourage positive social interactions as they proceed through school.

Acquisition of Social Knowledge

Social cognition, like cognitive growth, is a developmental process building upon new skills and insights as they are incorporated into the individual's thinking and behaviour. Through interaction with others, children learn such skills as listening, sharing, empathy, and morality. One of the more severe implications of vision loss is the resulting dependence upon others to mediate or intervene to ensure the person who is visually impaired has understood or is correctly interpreting information from the environment. This in itself is a complicated undertaking. Nesker-Simmons and Davidson (1992) stated:

> *It cannot be too strongly emphasized that, in order to take account of the unique developmental mode of young blind children, mediators must intervene much more than with sighted children. Paradoxically, in so doing, they run the risk of treating the children as 'different', thus violating the principles of normalization, and of making them dependent, reactive and passive, while intending to make them proactive and spontaneously curious. Mediation with blind children involves much higher levels of awareness, conscious planning and reflection, and systematic monitoring than with sighted children. (p. 33)*

Children with visual impairments frequently develop different conceptual understanding or experience delayed development relevant to social cognition. McAlpine (1992) found that children with visual acuities lower than 20/200 tended to have significant delays of four to five years in their perspective-taking ability, that is, their ability to understand that another individual could perceive a situation differently than they might. The importance of perspective taking is critical for such social skills as negotiation, conflict resolution, and empathy. Earlier in this text, it was also noted that social skills in such areas as these were highly correlated with popularity among school-age peers.

In relation to play, frequently cited as important to the development of social knowledge, Parsons (1986b) reported differences in both quantitative and qualitative patterns of play behaviour in young children with a visual impairment when compared to their peers who were fully sighted . The former spent less time in functional play activities (e.g., using a toy truck to haul sand) and more time involved in stereotypical play behaviours (e.g., holding the truck up-side-down and repeatedly rotating the wheels) than did their peers. Delays in perspective taking, perception of emotion, and appropriate use of social language involving the use of pronouns such as "I" and "me" are commonly reported in the research on children with visual impairments (McAlpine, 1992). How such delays influence social cognition are still not well understood.

Having a visual impairment can continue to restrict acquisition of social knowledge long after the preschool years. Corn and Bishop (1984) found the mean percentile scores of adolescents with a visual impairment on tests of practical knowledge acquisition to be significantly lower than those of their peers who were fully sighted. Furthermore, the lower scores of the children with low vision, when compared to subjects who were totally blind, suggests a tendency by parents and teachers to overlook the need for direct teaching of such information to children with low vision, as would be done for those who are totally blind. Children with low vision are often assumed to be able to acquire such knowledge through imitation just as their peers who are fully sighted do, however, this faulty assumption may result in children with low vision being at a greater risk for delays in social cognition than those children who are totally blind.

Those with a visual impairment are sometimes expected to automatically be able to accommodate their impairment by developing more effective use of their other senses. For many years it was assumed that those with a visual impairment could perceive the emotions of others solely from the verbal information they received. That is, they could interpret vocally expressed emotions. However, Minter, Hobson and Pring (1991) found that children who were congenitally blind were not as capable of recognizing vocally expressed emotions as were their peers who were sighted. Similar research by Matsuda (1984) stressed the importance of providing children with visual impairments with specific instruction in interpreting the verbal messages and moods of others. In addition to limiting the variety, frequency, and nature of social experiences from a very early age, a visual impairment also appears to interfere with the ability to interpret social messages.

Learning and Using Visual Cues

It is difficult to quantify the effect of vision loss or impaired vision on learning. Researchers have estimated that sixty to eighty percent of our learning is through information received visually. Adams and Faux have estimated that the average person receives over 60,000 visual messages every day. One's waking hours are spent both receiving and sending visual information. The amount of spontaneous learning resulting from observing and responding to visual information is immeasurable. Sonksen (1983) described the role of vision as "guardian of the personality, tutor of the senses, monitor of movement, and builder of concepts" (p. 92).

Limited access to both learning and using visual cues can be observed to detract from the social development of children with a visual impairment from a very early age. Interference with the reciprocal gazing between mother and child, characteristic of early parent-child interaction, is an example of the immediate negative effect vision loss has on social interaction. The tendency of those who are visually impaired not to make eye contact and the significant reduction in the frequency and variety of their facial expressions is frequently disconcerting to sighted individuals accustomed to the integral part these behaviours play in their communication. Hurt, Scott and McCroskey (1978) stressed the importance of such nonverbal communication to social interaction:

> *The use of eye movement is perceived as being one of the most meaningful cues in nonverbal communication, for it signals a willingness to interact and communicate. Direct eye contact with another in our culture normally communicates interest and attention. Conversely, lack of eye contact communicates lack of interest and attention. (p. 107)*

Lack of eye contact during interaction frequently creates a sense of uneasiness for participants. School children as young as six years of age have reported feelings of discomfort and annoyance when their classmate with a visual impairment did not look at them during conversations (MacCuspie, 1991). Frequently the sighted person responds to lack of eye contact by discontinuing the interaction as quickly as possible. Such reactions interfere with positive interactions between children who are visually impaired and their peers.

While eye contact is important, so is the coordination of speech and gestures.

> *[Face to face] interactions are rhythmic, cooperative activities, involving the complex coordination of speech and gesture. . . studies consistently find that successful interaction occurs when participants synchronize the rhythm of speech and gesture, while breakdowns occur in the absence of synchrony. (Mehan, 1978, p. 48)*

Such synchronization for those with a visual impairment is restricted, and for the totally blind perhaps even impossible, given the effect of vision loss on access to visual cues such as gestures and the feedback inherent in these cues. The complexity of human interaction and the importance of nonverbal communication create many opportunities for misinterpretation and misunderstanding during the process of the social interaction when one participant is visually impaired.

The vast number of social skills typical of a specific culture and their priority of importance in relation to social interaction is difficult to ascertain. Just as complex is the role vision plays in development and the subsequent consequences of impaired vision on psychological development and social interaction. Perception, "the process of sorting, coding, and organizing sensory data and concepts to make all the characteristics and operational functions fit together" is, according to Barraga, a "complex mental task" (1976, p. 41). It is an undertaking which each child learns to do in a unique way, referred to as the child's "cognitive style of learning" (Piaget, 1973). Vision plays an important role in helping a child coordinate and integrate the auditory and tactile stimuli from the environment, to imitate appropriate behaviour, and to learn concepts (Barraga, 1976; Scholl, 1986). Children with a visual impairment must rely increasingly upon senses other than vision as the degree of vision loss increases:

> *Totally blind individuals must rely on their other senses to obtain all the information about the world that they need, and partially sighted individuals need to make greater use of nonvisual information than sighted people. The role of perception in other areas of behavior is vast. This involvement is perhaps most obvious in locomotion, where the functions that nonvisual information must serve are reasonably clear. Perception is also critical in learning, and in cognitive and language development. Perception is important for socialization and personality development—a child must be able to perceive information about the wishes of other people in order to become socialized. (Warren, 1984, p. 49)*

The limited access to learning and using visual cues can be readily observed in a regular classroom where the student with a visual impairment may not respond to hand gestures beckoning her to be a partner, has difficulty locating desired peers in the cafeteria or on the playground, cannot observe or imitate the new games or activities popular among classmates, or does not respond to a friendly wave from across the room. Without formal activities to familiarize a blind child with all the children in a large class, the blind child can often be unaware of who his classmates are. Thus, visual information which comes through spontaneous interaction with one's environment is frequently inaccessible to children with severe visual impairments. The absence of this information can have significant negative consequences in relation to both their social and academic learning.

Feedback Through Nonverbal Communication

As mentioned in Chapter 2, children at 6 to 7 months of age can be observed using the person to whom they have a primary attachment as a social reference. In an unfamiliar situation they look at the adult's face to receive information relevant to the nature of the new situation. Nonverbal communication is a critical component of human interaction. Children soon learn to read the feelings of their peers by the expressions on their faces. As adults, nonverbal communication provides us with a wealth of information—how new ideas are being received by colleagues, how receptive the boss is to a request, how open to change a person may be, or how confident one feels. Of tremendous importance to social acceptance is the feedback we receive from others relevant to our behaviour. Appropriate behaviour, whether in the presence of adults or peers, usually receives positive responses such as smiles or nods of the head. Inappropriate behaviour, on the other hand, invariably elicits looks of disgust, annoyance, concern or perhaps disappointment.

Much of the nonverbal feedback available to sighted children is inaccessible to those who are visually impaired. This makes it difficult for them to develop and refine social interaction skills. They may not, for example, receive the nonverbal messages which encourage participation or friendship. Lack of response to such invitations by the child who is visually impaired is frequently interpreted by sighted peers as disinterest. Similarly, when students with a visual impairment behave inappropriately, for example, rock back and forth or press on their eyes, they do not see the responses such behaviour elicits on the faces of those who observe the behaviour. MacCuspie (1991) found that even in the early elementary school years, classmates were reluctant to make any verbal comments relevant to the inappropriate behaviour of their classmate who was visually impaired. Their response was more often to stare in bewilderment at the child or to discontinue any interaction. Furthermore, many teachers felt that speaking to the student with a visual impairment about inappropriate behaviour could emphasize the student's impairment or could hurt the child's feelings. In such situations, the inappropriate behaviour was ignored despite the fact that both teachers and peers found the behaviour disconcerting. By not receiving feedback which reinforces appropriate social behaviour and which discourages inappropriate actions, children with a visual impairment are significantly handicapped.

Physical Development and Agility

Although the gross motor milestones (e.g., crawling, sitting, walking) are usually delayed several months in children who are totally blind, those with low vision may demonstrate physical and gross motor development typical of children who are sighted (Fraiberg, 1977). However, children who are visually impaired are frequently less physically active because of such things as a hesitancy to move out into space, the limitations on the amount and timeliness of visual feedback, and the tendency of adults to be overprotective. DePauw (1981), in a review of the literature, concluded that, in general, students with a visual impairment have poor physical development characterized by reduced stamina and poor muscle tone and posture.

Playground activities in the early and middle elementary school years are often characterized by rough and tumble play, running, chasing, climbing, ball games, and skipping. In short, children are on the move. Although peers of a student with a visual impairment usually enjoy acting as a guide within the school building, on the playground they may find this responsibility interferes with opportunities for participation in some activities and slows down their pace (MacCuspie, 1991). For students with a visual impairment who travel independently on the playground, their level of physical agility must be comparable to their peers if they are to be routinely included in many activities. Consequently, the amount of social interaction, particularly on the playground, may be highly correlated with the students degree of physical fitness and agility.

As students with a visual impairment progress through school, activities requiring good physical development and agility are closely associated with friendship groups. Teenagers often get together after school to play various sports. Organized team sports play a prominent role in the social life of junior and senior high school students. Yet, even students with a visual impairment who can participate in some team sports at the elementary level find the advanced skill levels of team sports in junior and senior high beyond their visual abilities. Since team membership is often associated with group membership outside the gymnasium, as well as popularity among peers, students with a visual impairment may not have as many potential opportunities for inclusion in cliques or groups at this level. Again, the consequence of limited participation is frequently exclusion from the peer group.

Cultural Norms Associated with Communication Patterns

Closely associated with the acquisition of social knowledge are the cultural norms associated with social interaction and behaviour. The lack of eye contact during conversation with one who is visually impaired, as mentioned earlier, is often disconcerting for a sighted individual who has come to expect this response. Those who are visually impaired may unintentionally infringe on another's personal space by standing too close during conversations in order to gain better visual reference to the speaker. In the case of children who are totally blind, they may engage in a great deal of physical touching as they explore their environment. Learning the cultural limits of such touching is critical if the child is to avoid embarrassing peers or being avoided by them.

As well, within each culture there are specific roles (e.g., student, playmate, housewife) and associated behaviour patterns to learn. Scott (1969a) outlined the process of role learning in childhood and how visual impairment interferes with aspects of this process. First are the aspects of social roles the child is expected to learn during childhood, such as social and physical differentiations associated with gender. Children who are visually impaired, particularly those who are totally blind, have significant difficulty learning about the physiological differences between their bodies and those of the opposite sex (Scholl, 1986). This problem is compounded by the added restrictions vision loss places upon the ability to perceive and learn basic role traits and mannerisms associated with femininity and masculinity.

Another dimension of role learning is that associated with the basic knowledge required to act in a socially appropriate manner when interacting with others. The limitations visual impairment places upon imitation of appropriate behaviour are significant when one observes classmates' responses to the performance of some children who are visually impaired in integrated settings.

> *On the one hand, the child learns at least the basic rudiments of verbal behavior required by his role; on the other hand his physical conduct is inappropriate. This jarring discrepancy serves to heighten the perceived "differentness" between blind and sighted persons, thereby further isolating the blind youngster in his social contacts with others. (Scott, 1969a, p. 1043)*

Because the learning of these cultural norms is most often incidental, through imitation and routine participation in day-to-day activities, children with a visual impairment frequently have restricted access to essential aspects of their culture. Students with a visual impairment may also have limited access to other cultural information such as hairstyle, fashionable clothing, and gestures which are considered appropriate from the perspective of pupil culture. From an intervention standpoint, one must be a keen observer to note those aspects of a given culture which are being missed by the child with a visual impairment so that intervention to provide the missing information is devised.

Practice and Refinement of Interpersonal Skills

When considering the implications of visual impairment on social development and interaction discussed thus far, it is evident these children, by virtue of their impairment, face a significant risk of being neglected or rejected by their peers in an integrated setting. The result is frequently a significant reduction in the actual amount of peer interaction experienced by students with a visual impairment. Classroom teachers in a study done by Hoben and Lindstrom (1980) reported nearly half of these students spent most of their unstructured time alone.

Interaction with peers is essential to social learning and vital to the development of appropriate social skills. Through interaction with peers a child learns to share, perceive the viewpoints of others, mediate conflict, participate in conversations and activities, and to develop friendships. All of these behaviours require tremendous amounts of practice and experimentation if the child is to understand how to interact effectively. If children who are visually impaired are placed in integrated settings without structured programming and routine monitoring of their social interaction and acceptance, it is probable they will experience difficulties associated with social acceptance. It can become a vicious circle. The child with a visual impairment enters school with inadequate social skills which limit social exchanges and active participation. While unstructured time is spent alone or in limited interaction, other children who are socially involved for the major part of the day are practising and refining their social skills. Absence of opportunities to have such practice serves to increase the social gap between the child who is visually impaired and classmates. Thus, it can be speculated that one of the most severe consequences for children with a visual impairment who have not been well accepted by their peers is the compounding effect of the ongoing reduction in their opportunities to practice and refine critical social skills.

Studies of the correlation between the sociometric status of students with a visual impairment and the length of time classmates have known these students support this speculation. In separate studies Eaglestein (1975) and Goupil and Comeau (1983) found correlations between the length of time a student with a visual impairment was known by classmates and the scores on scales determining the degree of liking and willingness to work with the student. Results indicated that the longer students with a visual impairment were known by classmates, the less likely their peers were to like or to be willing to work with them. Such findings should not lead the reader to believe that early integration should be avoided but rather should emphasize the critical importance of timely programming and routine monitoring of the social interaction and acceptance of students with a visual impairment.

Perceptions Associated with Mannerisms

Children who are blind or who have a severe vision loss may develop stereotypic behaviours, often referred to in the literature as blindisms or mannerisms in the literature. These are repetitive, idiosyncratic actions such as body rocking, light gazing, eye pressing, head motions, or arm flapping. A number of theories as to the cause of mannerisms have been proposed. Olson (1986) suggested that they may act as an outlet for the release of energy which would normally be used in seeing, provide external stimulation when the child is not active, act as pleasurable stimulation, act as a substitute for satisfying human relationships, or result from faulty neurological development.

> *Regardless of their cause, mannerisms generally become established during the first few years of life, are very difficult to extinguish, and have a negative effect upon social interaction and acceptance by one's peers (Scott, 1969a).*

In a public school setting, children who frequently indulge in such mannerisms are perceived by their peers to act differently from other children (MacCuspie, 1991). Classmates feel these behaviours are undesirable and strange. They come to believe that these "weird" actions are a natural consequence of having a visual impairment. Mannerisms can interfere with social interaction in a number of ways. For example, a child may be reluctant to either initiate or continue a conversation with someone who is actively involved in what appears to be some form of self-stimulation or inappropriate behaviour. Often a classmate will be hesitant to maintain an association with a student who is perceived to be "acting weird." When a child is exhibiting a mannerism such as rocking, he/she is often "in a world of her/his own" and seemingly uninterested in social exchange. It is not uncommon for peer initiated interaction to be rebuffed in such circumstances. Furthermore, teachers frequently respond to mannerisms by ignoring them. Classmates may be confused when a teacher who routinely addresses inappropriate behaviour in other children overlooks what is perceived to be inappropriate behaviour in the student with a visual impairment.

Distinct facial Features or Appearance

As mentioned in Chapter 2, physical attractiveness is correlated with popularity. A distinct difference in appearance (e.g., the pale complexion and white hair associated with albinism) is frequently viewed negatively by children, even at the early elementary school level. Many children with a visual impairment have distinct facial features specific to their eye condition. Strabismus (i.e., divergence in gaze), nystagmus (i.e., involuntary rapid eye movement), corneal scarring, or sunken eye sockets are associated with some eye conditions and may contribute to the child with a visual impairment appearing different from others. As well, the body posture and gait of children with a severe visual impairment is often different from or awkward in comparison to that of their peers. It is difficult to determine the extent to which such variables interfere with social interaction and acceptance of children with visual impairments, but in many schools being different is not highly correlated with either social acceptance or popularity. It is probable that the physical appearance of some children with a visual impairment increases the likelihood that classmates may be reluctant to interact with them. This limited interaction makes it difficult for relationships involving the child with a visual impairment to progress from an acquaintance to a friendship. Without formal instruction and open discussion of issues relevant to having a visual impairment, many myths (e.g., visual impairment is a punishment for past sins) and misconceptions associated with blindness continue to exist.

Negative Attitudes Toward Those with Disabilities

As mentioned in earlier chapters, the real beliefs and feelings one may hold in regard to those who are visually impaired are frequently not the positive assumptions essential to social acceptance by one's peers. If the integration of students with a visual impairment is to influence a change in these negative attitudes, classmates must have experiences which challenge the myths and misconceptions traditionally associated with those who are visually impaired. Mead (1934) believed that the self is given meaning through the process of interaction as a result of the attitudes expressed by significant others toward it. Therefore, one's self-concept develops in relation to the meanings others construct and reflect toward one, both explicitly and implicitly, during social interaction.

Children with a visual impairment learn from a very early age that having a visual impairment is problematic for their parents, teachers, and playmates.

Our language is full of negative images associated with visual impairment—"poor vision", "can't do it because you are blind", "can't read or write as fast because you are visually impaired", "normal people have normal vision." There is a real danger that children with a visual impairment come to believe the impairment is the most prominent attribute of their being and furthermore, this attribute is a negative one. Thus, their potential to develop a positive self-concept and high self-esteem is threatened.

As well, feedback received during social interaction may be inaccurately interpreted by those who are visually impaired or inappropriately provided by those without disabilities. Scott (1969b) discussed the confusion created within the child who is visually impaired when adults, in particular, are overgenerous with praise for even the most trivial accomplishment. This results in the child either considering herself/himself exceptionally talented or considering the blind to be particularly incompetent if such insignificant actions result in unwarranted praise. In either case, the social consequences are apt to be undesirable.

> *Self-images are formed from beliefs about ourselves that are integrated with those that others hold of us. Each blind and visually impaired child needs to feel that he is a worthy and contributing member of the family and the peer group, as well as a unique individual with special talents and abilities. The visual impairment is part of the self and must be incorporated into the total self-image, but it is only one of the many attributes, feelings, and emotions. Exaggerated feelings about the limitations imposed by the impairment give it a larger role than it deserves. It is hoped that the child will come to believe that opportunities are opened because of his abilities and not closed because of the impairment. (Swallow & Huebner, 1987, p. 29)*

If students with a visual impairment who are integrated in regular classrooms view themselves as inappropriate workmates or playmates for their peers, it is obvious they will be reluctant to make a concerted effort to promote their own social acceptance or interaction.

Interaction Stress

Communication involves an exchange between at least two individuals. When there are perceived, significant differences between these individuals the act of natural and spontaneous communication may be altered to the extent that the individuals are unable to comfortably accommodate their differences. As we have seen, there are many complicating variables present in the interaction between a child with a visual impairment and a classmate. Davis (1961) suggested that an impairment poses four basic risks to social interaction. They are:

- the tendency for the impairment to become the exclusive focal point of the exchange
- the creation of a discrepancy between real feelings about the impairment and the pressure to respond in an appropriate manner
- the struggle to resolve this discrepancy by assimilating the two feelings which may then result in patronizing or condescending thoughts or comments (e.g., How strange someone who is blind could be so capable!)
- the extent to which the impairment is perceived to interfere with the natural and spontaneous initiation of an activity in which both parties can freely participate.

When students with a visual impairment are integrated in a regular classroom they and their peers must have the opportunity to overcome these aspects of interaction stress. Real social acceptance cannot develop until classmates have had the opportunity to "really get to know" the student who is visually impaired and understand the nature of the eye condition and its implications for learning and social interaction.

When Smith and Smith (1983) studied the social behaviour of teenage students who attended a residential school for the blind, they found the social behaviours of the students with a visual impairment were typical of those found in any junior or senior high school. Social interaction was spontaneous and natural, characterized by friendships and boy-girl relationships. Additionally, students gathered in groups associated with specific interests such as sports, music, or other recreational pursuits. Their social exchange was not hampered by the knowledge of the presence of impairment or mannerisms. Despite the fact that many of these students, in all probability, had some delays or gaps in social or cognitive development, among friends there was the support needed to accommodate such shortcomings. Interaction stress was obviously significantly reduced and participants were able to move beyond the initial barriers to positive interaction and to develop real friendships. Most importantly, in this social environment students had the opportunity to practice and refine the social skills essential to effective human communication. This should not lead the reader to believe that residential placements create more effective social environments for children, but rather to understand that the child with a visual impairment is not necessarily asocial or lacking in social skills. What must be addressed in integrated settings is how to enhance the social acceptance of those who have traditionally been segregated from the usual social environments of childhood

Contextual Factors

The social environment in schools is a complex one. Therefore, the acceptance of children with a visual impairment will obviously be a multifaceted phenomenon. There are conceivably hundreds of aspects of a given situation which may influence, either positively or negatively, the perceptions constructed by individuals who are fully sighted and the degree to which students with a visual impairment are accepted by their peers. Unique circumstances within a given school (e.g., the congestion of the playground and resulting safety considerations for the student with a visual impairment) may have a negative influence on the child's acceptance. There are also variables which appear to be common to many schools (e.g., the expectation that children who are different from their peers will be less acceptable to their classmates). Sometimes a variable which appears to be particularly potent at one school will be unremarkable in a different school environment. The complexity of social activity in schools makes it difficult to isolate single variables which can be identified as consistently positive or negative influences on the social acceptance of children.

Nonetheless, some aspects of school environments frequently appear to contribute to or detract from the acceptance and interaction of many students, not just those with a disability. If students, for example, are unable to complete tasks within the assigned time, they have fewer opportunities to participate in the social interaction which routinely occurs among other students as they complete one task and prepare for the next. When these students are routinely unavailable to participate in such "between task socializing," they may have difficulty joining in on occasions when they are available. Similarly, in classrooms where children are seated in group arrangements the frequency of interaction among students may be significantly higher than in those classrooms where students are sitting in rows at individual desks. The potential implications of such variables on the social acceptance and interaction of children in general, are shared by students with a visual impairment who are integrated in the regular classroom.

There is clearly a multiplicity of contextual issues at play as students with a visual impairment interact with their classmates. To facilitate discussion of such contextual issues, they have been grouped into categories primarily relevant to students with a visual impairment, classmates of these students, teachers, classroom environments, the structure of playgrounds, and administrative arrangements.

Students with a visual impairment will obviously vary in age, gender, physical attractiveness, social competence, physical agility, maturity in relation to peers, personality (e.g., extrovert, assertive, sense of humour, friendliness, self-esteem), openness to discuss visual impairment, academic performance, level of independence, commitment to the peer group, and in numerous other ways. These attributes of the children, captured at a given point in time, can be seen to contribute to or detract from their social acceptance and interaction with peers. An extroverted child, regardless of the presence or absence of a disability, who routinely participates in group discussions may be more readily included in classroom activities and sought out for a partner than one who frequently sits by himself and rarely contributes to class discussions. Thus, the social acceptance of students with a visual impairment is not merely a function of being visually impaired or of the child's level of social competence, but a complex process inextricably part of the nature of the social environment and the personality of the participant.

Just as children who are visually impaired present a variety of characteristics, so do their classmates. There are children of different ages, gender, ethnic backgrounds, religious affiliations, academic abilities, physical prowess, temperaments, and socio-economic levels. Some children may be more committed to the rules of pupil culture than others; some children may be more willing to include a student with a visual impairment than others. Students who are self-confident and excel in a variety of areas have been found to be less threatened by accomplishments of students with a visual impairment and less resentful of the special attention these students may be perceived to receive than are students without such skills. As well, girls, perhaps because they are socialized to nurture, frequently seem to be more tolerant and inclusive toward students with a disability than are boys (MacCuspie, 1991).

Issues relevant to the teachers of students with a visual impairment may also have a positive or negative influence upon the degree of social acceptance and interaction experienced by these children. Teachers vary in the degree to which they are supportive of integration, to which they are willing to accommodate certain disabilities, and to which they are able to adjust the program for the child rather than vice versa. As well, teachers differ in their willingness to undertake the additional work which may be associated with accommodating a student with a visual impairment, their degree of comfort in having other adults (e.g., teacher assistants or specialist teachers) in their classroom, and their skill in incorporating new teaching strategies to enhance the performance of the student with a visual impairment. Teacher empathy is an aspect of the school environment which appears to contribute to a positive experience for students with a visual impairment in an integrated setting. In fact, for all students:

> *Teacher empathy is the core skill that underlies special teaching . . . empathy goes far beyond the verbal exchange and is reflected in how the teacher manages instruction, organizes the school environment, responds to the feelings of the pupils, and is able to be calm, warm and show affection. We all went through the age processes, but, frequently we have lost the capacity to reactivate the pupil's view in ourselves. (Morse, Ardissone, Macdonald & Pasick, 1980, p. 20)*

A fourth category of contextual variables includes those associated with the organization and physical layout of the classroom, as well as the learning environment created within it. As mentioned earlier in the chapter, certain group seating arrangements increase the frequency of interaction and inclusion of the student with a visual impairment. As well, such factors as class size, the strictness relative to communication within the classroom, and the type of arrangements developed to assist the student with a visual impairment (e.g., "pull-out" versus "in class" assistance) may also contribute to the degree of acceptance extended and frequency of interaction available to students with a visual impairment. When students with a visual impairment are removed from the class to receive special instruction, classmates are frequently suspicious of or curious about these private tutorial lessons. Even teachers may tend to renounce responsibility for the student's learning while he/she is absent from the class.

Programs which specifically promote the acceptance and active participation of students with disabilities in both the social and the academic life of the school are becoming more prominent. Co-operative learning is one instructional approach which appears to provide some potential for effectively addressing some of the issues relevant to social integration. In comparison with individualistic and competitive learning practices, co-operative learning appears to promote higher self-esteem for all students, including those with disabilities (Johnson & Johnson, 1984).

For students with a visual impairment, classrooms which promote more cooperative approaches to learning are also those which increase the opportunities for social interaction of the student. They provide greater opportunities to demonstrate the student's abilities and minimize the emphasis on the disability and its restrictions. The restrictions imposed by an impairment are frequently emphasized in a competitive environment where only the best accomplishments are valued. In an integrated setting, if peer relationships are to be a constructive influence on the affective development of children, educators and parents must orchestrate learning environments that promote feelings of acceptance and not those of alienation.

Contextual factors associated with the structure of the playground also influence the social acceptance and interaction of students with a visual impairment. There are aspects of pupil culture which have immediate consequences for the social acceptance and interaction of students with a visual impairment. For example, there must be a selection of activities in which children with a visual impairment can successfully participate. Other variables which influence the inclusion of these students are such things as the safety of the playground for a student with a visual impairment, the congestion of the playground, the time spent on the playground, and the size and layout of the playground.

The final category of issues are those associated with administrative aspects of the school, in general, and the administration of integration, in particular, which may influence the social acceptance and interaction of students with a visual impairment. The leadership role of the principal in creating a climate conducive to the social integration of students with disabilities is crucial. Researchers have consistently shown that those beliefs and programs routinely discussed by and attended to by the principal are those which are effectively implemented in schools (Sergiovanni, 1984). The principal must involve teachers in the development of school level policy or plans for integration and expose them to the philosophical and pragmatic issues inherent within the concept of integration.

It is clear there is a need for integration to be addressed in the following ways:

- as a school issue,
- as an innovation to education which requires preparation of teachers,
- as an approach to learning which necessitates a team effort,
- as a process which has serious implications for emotional development of integrated children, and
- as a process which has the potential to enhance the learning environment for all children.

The absence of a team approach to integration frequently results in inconsistency in both implementation of a child's program and interaction with the student. The implications of this are particularly evident when the teacher assigned the student is left to single-handedly design and implement programs without the assistance and support of fellow educators and parents. Without a team approach to integration, the role of teacher assistants is frequently misunderstood and these paraprofessionals may inadvertently take on responsibilities which are inappropriate. The assignment of a teacher assistant who is constantly with the student with a visual impairment may interfere with the spontaneous interaction between this student and other classmates. Too frequently assigned assistants take over the instructional responsibilities of the teacher removing the child from the group for individual instruction. This further limits the amount of peer interaction experienced by the student with a visual impairment.

The complexities inherent within the many contextual variables discussed in this chapter can be overwhelming. The same factor which exerts a positive influence in one situation might have a negative effect upon the inclusion of another student in a different situation. Single variables are difficult to isolate as constants relative to their effect on the acceptance or rejection of a student. However, each aspect of the context, inextricably linked with hundreds of others within the environment and to the interaction of its participants, appear to have varying degrees of importance as people interpret and respond to the social acceptance and interaction of students with a visual impairment.

In this chapter we have explored the potential barriers to social acceptance and interaction encountered by students with a visual impairment. These barriers are complex. Some are associated with the effects vision loss has on cognitive, physical, and affective development and may be overcome or accommodated through timely intervention and training for children with a visual impairment and their parents. Some are associated with aspects of the individual with a visual impairment that cannot be changed (e.g., appearance). Still others are associated with those who are fully sighted and their capacity to develop a more inclusive social environment, one that promotes the positive acceptance of those with an impairment.

In the next section of this book, the findings of a study which focused upon the social acceptance and interaction of elementary students with a visual impairment will be discussed. The findings of this study may help to clarify how an integrated setting can unintentionally become a hostile environment for students with a visual impairment when integration is not implemented with careful attention to the implications it has for teachers and students. In the final section of this book, suggestions and guidelines to enhance the social integration of students with a visual impairment will be presented. With an understanding of the complexities involved in the integration process, readers will be able to adapt the potential solutions recommended to their specific circumstances.

Section II

A Qualitative Research Study on the Social Integration of Children with a Visual Impairment

4

Pupil Culture and Its Implications for the Social Integration of Students with a Visual Impairment

Introduction

Social acceptance is an outcome of positive social interaction and meaningful participation in the routine activities of the school day. Programs which have attempted to improve the social acceptance of children with disabilities have traditionally focused on the social skill level of the child with the disability. For example, a child with a visual impairment might receive specific training in directing gaze toward the face of the speaker or in strategies to use when attempting to join a group of children who are playing. Regardless of the disability involved, these programs have had limited success in making long-term improvements in social acceptance. Programs which attempt to increase the understanding and awareness of all participants in the social environment as well as teaching social skills are proving to be much more effective. In a social environment which encourages the positive acceptance of difference and attempts to understand the implications of an impairment on both learning and social integration, all children will thrive.

Educators and parents cannot be content to function at a "blame the victim" level where they assume the child's social isolation is primarily a consequence of immature or inappropriate behaviours or social skills. It is essential to examine the social environment in which children with disabilities must interact and identify those aspects which contribute to and detract from their social acceptance. To provide the reader with a perspective on how the social environment influences social acceptance, the next three chapters will focus on the research recently completed by the author. This research investigated the role pupil and school culture played in the social acceptance and interaction of five elementary school children with a visual impairment who were integrated in regular classrooms in their local public schools.

The Study

The study explored the social environment of the elementary school and the process of social interaction and acceptance between children with a visual impairment and their sighted peers. A multi-site case study approach was employed. Five classrooms in four different schools located in two Canadian provinces were chosen for the study. Five visually impaired participants, four with low vision and one who was totally blind, in grades one through six, were randomly chosen from an identified population of approximately 44 children. These were children who had a visual acuity of 20/200 or less, were without additional disabilities, were achieving at grade level, and did not demonstrate behavioral problems.

Participant observation, interviews, and the study of various documents were employed in the collection and analysis of data. Approximately five months were spent observing at the schools, one month in each classroom with an integrated student. Data was collected from the following sources:

- full day observation in five classrooms where a student with a visual impairment was enrolled
- both formal and informal interviews with students with a visual impairment, five to eight of their classmates, their teachers, itinerant teachers for the visually impaired, principals and parents
- analysis of documents available at the site (e.g., newsletters, individualized education programs, report cards, procedure manuals) and those relevant to integration policy published by provincial Departments of Education.

From these data, basic assumptions of pupil and school culture relating to friendship, acceptance, and peer interaction were identified and examined in relation to the social acceptance and interaction of students with a visual impairment.

The Students With A Visual Impairment

All five students with a visual impairment in this study were enrolled in regular classrooms and received two to five hours of individual instruction from an itinerant teacher for the visually impaired. Despite these commonalities, there was tremendous variability in the situations and circumstances in the lives of these children. The following information is provided to give the reader a sense of the individuals in the study.

Peter. Peter was the eldest of three children and lived with his parents on a small farm. He travelled by bus to attend a Grade 4 class in the nearby village. Peter was a co-operative, diligent, ten year old student with a serious but friendly manner. His diagnosis was optic nerve hypoplasia with light perception in the left eye, a visual acuity of 20/400, and a field restriction in the right eye.

Lisa. Lisa was the elder of two children living with her mother and brother on the outskirts of a small community. She had albinism and displayed many of the associated characteristics (i.e., white hair, pale skin, nystagmus, a visual acuity of 20/400). As a student, Lisa's teachers described her as talkative, outgoing, capable, and assertive bordering on aggressive. She was six years old and was enrolled in a Grade one class with her twenty-eight classmates.

Tony. Tony, age eight, was the third of four children. His mother had been married three times and she and the children lived in a trailer with her third husband. Tony travelled by bus to the nearby town where he was enrolled in Grade 3 in an overcrowded school. As a student Tony was enthusiastic, interested, and actively participated in every aspect of the school program. He was totally blind as a result of retinopathy of prematurity.

Jamie. Jamie, age ten, and his older sister lived with their mother in a townhouse in a suburb of a small city. His visual impairment, caused by optic atrophy, was not diagnosed until he was nearly four years of age. Jamie's visual impairment could not be detected from his appearance. In addition to a visual acuity of 20/200, he had poor colour vision and difficulties with night vision. He was enrolled in Grade 5 at a large, neighbourhood school where he participated in all aspects of his school program.

Charles. Charles and his younger sister lived with their parents in a suburban area about one mile from his school. Charles was a year older than most of his twelve year old, Grade 6 classmates. As a result of retinopathy of prematurity, Charles was blind in his left eye and had a visual acuity of 20/400 with restricted fields in the right eye. Teachers described Charles as a shy but diligent student. His awkward gait and poor coordination limited his active participation in many playground activities.

The Social Environments of Schools

The importance of time as a central organizing principle of the everyday world of schooling is often overlooked as a unique aspect of school. Time plays a critical role in the type and range of curriculum covered in a given classroom. In the five classrooms in this study, time tended to condition and pattern the types of interaction in which children participated. In conjunction with other structuring factors such as the proximity of the teacher, the negotiated rules of the specific class being attended, or the schedule for a particular day, time created opportunities for and limitations upon pupil interaction. At one site the time required at the beginning of each day to collect milk and lunch money provided an opportunity for interaction among children sitting in proximity to one another. At another site the 15-minute morning recess was the only time the entire school population was gathered simultaneously on the playground. Therefore, the structuring effect of time was important to the kinds of interaction which children experienced.

The vast amount of time available to children to interact with their peers was remarkable. Opportunities for social exchange exist when children gathered in the school yard waiting to be admitted to the school; as they entered and removed their outside clothing; as they awaited the singing of "O Canada" and the morning announcements; as the teacher attended to "housekeeping tasks" such as collecting milk or lunch money; as they got out and put away books and other learning materials before and after each lesson; as part of class discussions; as they worked on an assigned task in small groups; as they filed in line-ups to and from the bathroom, the water fountain, or other classrooms; at morning and noon hour recesses; as they ate their lunch; as they gathered their things at the end of the day; and as they left the school to walk or travel by bus to their homes. Although the total time available for interaction was determined to some extent by the rules regulating when interaction was permitted, as well as the degree to which these rules were enforced in specific classrooms and schools, it appeared that the major part of the school day was conducive to social exchange among children. Even during those times when interaction was prohibited, for example, when students were instructed to work independently or when the teacher was talking, non-verbal exchanges occurred.

Time also shaped the relationships and hence the interactions of children in two crucial respects. First, the stage in the school year had some relevance to the composition of play groups. Early in the new school year, play groups or friendship patterns were not well established. However, within several months, most children played exclusively with classmates, that is, those from their classroom. Second, time was relevant to the types of activities in which children participated, as well as the types of relationships created. Peer interaction at the grade one level differed from that at the grade six level in relation to the duration of friendships, boy-girl relationships, and the types of activities in which they participated. Additionally, activities on the playground varied from season to season (e.g., coasting and sliding on the ice in January, skipping and baseball in the spring).

Children participated in a variety of types of interactions with their peers. Classroom interactions were characterized by quiet talk or use of "inside voices" (i.e., not the yelling and screaming which characterized playground interaction) and limited movement from place to place. On the playground interactions more often involved some form of physical contact such as jostling, pushing, holding hands, or huddling in small exclusive groups. Children "on the run" from one area to another appeared to be a hallmark of playground behaviour.

On the playground interactions varied in relation to the activity in which the child was involved. When participating in pretend play, actors took on the role and personalities of their favourite characters, such as Ghost Busters and

Teenage Mutant Ninja Turtles, or the mother, father, or "kid," if playing house. Within the school as well, activities tended to influence the nature of interaction among children. During some activities children were permitted to move about the classroom and could more easily assemble with their "best friends" than during formal lessons in which independent work was required. The formalities of social exchanges such as turn taking, using manners, and sharing were also generally monitored and commented upon by teachers within the confines of their classroom. On the playground this was rarely the case.

The Concept of School Culture

During the past decade the "effective schools movement" has placed considerable emphasis on school culture. Purkey and Smith (1982) defined the school's culture as "a structure, process, and climate of values and norms that channel staff and students in the direction of successful teaching and learning" (p. 64).

School culture, the "unseen supervisor" was viewed by Alfonso (1986) as "something that helps keep teachers on target, that teaches them how to behave, establishes standards, values, and sanctions, and which provides guidance and validation for one's work" (p. 5). Schein (1985) defined culture as follows:

> *A pattern of basic assumptions—invented, discovered, or developed by a given group as it learns to cope with its problems of external adaptation and internal integration—that has worked well enough to be taught to new members as the correct way to perceive, think, and feel in relation to those problems. (p. 9)*

Schein differentiated among three levels of culture. At the first level are artifacts. These include such things as physical arrangements of the organization, language, social atmosphere, and conspicuous actions of its members. Values are at the second level. They serve the moral function of the organization's members and distinguish between "what is" and "what ought to be." Artifacts and values, however, are merely manifestations of the culture. At the third level, "the essence of culture," are the basic assumptions of the organization. Schein (1985) stated:

> *The term culture should be reserved for the deeper level of basic assumptions and beliefs that are shared by members of an organization that operate unconsciously, and that define in a basic taken-for-granted fashion an organization's view of itself and its environment. These assumptions and beliefs are learned responses to a group's problems of internal integration. They come to be taken-for-granted because they solve these problems repeatedly and reliably. This deeper level of assumptions is to be distinguished from the 'artifacts' and 'values' that are the manifestations or surface levels of the culture, but not the essence of the culture. (pp. 6-7)*

Thus, Schein (1985) developed the concept of culture beyond the superficial level of climate, ethos, or values. As well, his concept of culture emphasized the examination of social units within the host culture, such as teacher culture or pupil culture. In this study, an attempt was made to identify cultural assumptions which were associated with the acceptance and interaction of students with a visual impairment.

Assumptions of Pupil Culture Relevant to Social Integration

Eleven basic assumptions of pupil culture relevant to the acceptance and interaction of children were identified from participant-observation notes and interview transcripts. Codes were created for emerging themes, insights, specific research questions, key concepts and common interaction patterns. As patterns and interrelationships emerged, the links among the concepts were specified and refined. Triangulation, i.e., cross-checking the accuracy of data among several sources, was used to confirm findings and substantiate the basic cultural assumptions. These assumptions, as with any cultural assumption, are implicit in the pupils' actions and words — they are not explicit "rules" the children state.

Pupil Assumption 1: *In school, children ought to play and associate with their "best friends."*

"Best friends" are nice to one another, always play together, don't leave to join other groups, hang around together, and are fun to be with. There is a definite distinction between "best" and "okay" friends. "Okay friends" only play with each other now and then, don't usually hang around together, are not as nice to one another as are "best friends," and sometimes argue with or "act snobby" toward one another. "Okay friends" are the ones a child chooses to associate with when "best friends" are not available.

Children who are "not friends" fall into two groups. In the first group are children who hurt other children, tease or are mean to others, don't hang around with one another, talk back or won't talk at all to another child, and often won't give permission for other children to play with them. The second group of children classified as "not friends" are children whom others don't know very well.

The following excerpt from an interview with a grade 5 student typifies the way children categorized their classmates: [Note: In interview excerpts, the letter "I" is the interviewer and the letter "R" the respondent.]

I: *What's the difference between "best friends" and "okay friends"?*
R: *Um, I..I talk to my best friends a lot more.*
I: *Your "best friends" you talk to more.*
R: *Yes.*
I: *What other differences?*

R: *Um..ah..well, these guys [pointing to names of "best friends"] I've never really got mad at but some of these people ["okay friends"] I've lost my temper with.*

I: *Okay, so you don't really get mad at your "best friends." Tell me about this group of kids who are not your friends.*

R: *Darren, I got in a fight with him cuz he was calling me names and everything. And I, I've tried my hardest to be so nice to him. And he started to do that and I just lost my temper. Matthew, he, I don't know about Matthew. And Wendell, he's changed. Like before he'd, he..he picks on my brother a lot. He doesn't pick on me, but when he does on my brother it eats me up inside.*

I: *Umhmm. Okay. And Michelle?*

R: *Um, I don't know. She..not a lot of people like her. I don't know why. [classmate, Grade 5]*

In class a "best friend" is chosen for a partner whenever possible. If a student doesn't have a "best friend" a partner must be chosen from the children who are "left over" after the "best friends" have paired off. On the playground, "best friends" play with one another and travel about together. Thus, "best friends" routinely seek each other's companionship.

Only one of the five students with a visual impairment observed in this study had a mutual "best friend," that is, someone whom he spontaneously identified as a "best friend" and was, in turn, considered by this classmate to be his "best friend." However, both of these boys were considered by their classmates to be outside "the group." One other child with a visual impairment was named in an interview with a classmate as a "best friend" but interaction on the playground, in the classroom, and outside school hours was infrequent. Four of the students who were visually impaired did have "okay friends" and were generally considered by their classmates as an "okay friend," that is, one with whom a child chooses to associate when "best friends" are not available.

The perceptions associated with a "best friend" were different for the children who were visually impaired than for their classmates. Children who were visually impaired consistently emphasized two significant criteria for friends—"they don't make fun of my eyesight" and "if I have problems they'll help me out." Thus, these students did not seem to identify "best friends" on the basis of frequent or routine interaction. In fact, three of the children with a visual impairment appeared to struggle with the concept of "best friends." This was particularly evident when they were asked to differentiate between "best friends" and "okay friends." They were less specific and more uncertain about the nature of friendship than were their peers. Whether they lacked experiences with childhood friendships or their visual limitations resulted in a different experience, their verbalized perception of friendship was different from that of their classmates.

In general, classmates of the students who were visually impaired perceived them to either have best friends outside the classroom group or not to have any. They did not report the students who were visually impaired to have the same kind of "best friends" as they themselves had. For example, when asked to name the friends of the student who was visually impaired, one classmate reported, "Well, there's me and Marla, and Nat, and Paul. He doesn't really have best, best friends, but he has good friends." As mentioned, "good" or "okay friends" were more akin to acquaintances and were the neutral ground between "best friends" and those who were not one's friends.

Pupil Assumption 2: ***To be part of a group a child ought to be able to do what the other children are doing.***

There are two components involved in being able to do what the other children are doing. First, a child must be able to participate actively and independently in the activity (e.g., skipping, playing marbles, soccer, or baseball). Second, a certain level of competence must be evident. Students who do not meet these criteria will be ostracized or, in unusual circumstances, patronized.

For students with a visual impairment there were two major aspects to consider in relation to this assumption. First, they had to have sufficient visual efficiency to participate in the specific task. There were some activities which were inappropriate for students with a severe visual impairment (e.g., copying notes from the board, playing dodge ball). Second, they had to have a level of skill acceptable to their playmates so as not to detract from the enjoyment of other participants, particularly if there was competition involved. In the classroom, for the most part, the five students with a visual impairment could do what their classmates were doing. Yet, there were two aspects of competence which were noticeably different. First, the rate at which they read and wrote was slower than that of their peers. Three of the children required almost twice the amount of time as their peers to independently complete the tasks assigned. Second, the appearance of the written work of four of the children was noticeably different from that of their classmates in size, legibility, and style. In general, it had the appearance of work produced by much younger children. In many cases, students who were sighted tended to judge the work of their classmate with a visual impairment as inferior to that of other students. Furthermore, they were not perceived to be doing the same thing as their classmates when they used different materials (e.g., large print books, texts on tape); hence, they were frequently viewed as less desirable group members. However, few tasks were either inordinately difficult or technically impossible for students with a visual impairment.

On the playground, three of the students who were visually impaired experienced major difficulties participating in the typical activities of their sighted classmates (e.g., chase games, ball games) because the majority of the games were beyond their levels of competence. Additionally, they experienced difficulties with the level of noise and congestion on the playgrounds. They tended to remain in a particular spot (e.g., on the swings) or to pace back and forth in a quieter, less congested area. In general, their physical agility and skill levels were far below those of their peers. However, two of the children with a visual impairment were not noticeably less competent on the playground than their peers. That is, they enjoyed and could actively participate in the majority of the activities involving their classmates because they were at a similar skill level.

The perceptions children with a visual impairment had of their incompetence in some activities appeared to have a direct effect upon when and what activities they would attempt to join. In the following excerpt from an interview with Jamie, a grade five student who was visually impaired, it is obvious he had learned that a certain level of competence was a prerequisite to his participation with peers:

I: *I noticed on the playground you don't seem to have one or two kids whom you always hang around with?*

R: *I know.*

I: *It's different each day. Can you tell me about that?*

R: *Because like, sometimes, it depends really, cuz like, sometimes other kids are having too much fun, and on the off chance some persons aren't having fun, I just walk around with him. And on the other days, if someone, if the person I hung around with the day before is with someone else and the other guys are not with anyone else, that's when I'll hang around with them.*

I: *When you say they're having too much fun, if a group is having too much fun, do you join with that group?*

R: *Well, it depends what they're doing, cuz if they're having too much fun playing catch or something, and they don't think I'm that good at it, then I don't, I don't bother with it. Cuz I don't like getting into arguments with other people...for no reason. [Grade 5]*

In addition to concerns about their level of competence, some of the students with a visual impairment also had concerns about their safety in particular situations. The following excerpt was typical:

I: *When we were talking about what you liked to do at recess and noon hour, you said you preferred the swings because some of the other games were too dangerous. What games do you think are too dangerous for you?*

R: *And some I can't even do!*

I: *Oh, okay tell me about the ones you think are too dangerous and the ones you can't even do.*

R: *Like monkey bar tag, I cannot play that. It's dangerous. Cuz I can't even get up on the monkey bars and it, and if, and since I can't, I might run around the ground if I want to play. And someone could go "oomp" and kick me right in the eye and then knock my sight out forever. See that's why I hate, I don't like the monkey bars.*

I: *So monkey bar tag is a game that is too dangerous. Are there any others that are too dangerous?*

R: *Baseball, because, like maybe if I'm trying to hit that ball, the ball might come and hit me right in there [points to eyes] and I might not see it.*

I: *Now tell me about some of the games you can't do?*

R: *Tag, I'm not fast enough for it. And baseball, like if we were playing down in the field, may have a real game going, and I was, say I was up, and I hit the ball, and say I was running, but the pitcher might be faster than me, see?*

I: *Ummhm.*

R: *And he could go boomp, and say, "You're out." See, see, I need more speed and more, better sight. [Peter, Grade 4]*

During the five months of observation of children with a visual impairment, it became evident that they had restricted access to information relevant to both their level of competence and that of their peers. For example, all four pupils who used print were known for their large, "messy" penmanship. They perceived themselves to have inferior skills in this area, but interestingly, none was aware of other children in the class with similar difficulties, that is, poor penmanship. Such lack of knowledge was common, both in the classroom and on the playground, and it seemed to contribute to a belief by children with a visual impairment that sighted people were "super beings," making it difficult for them to perceive their "own errors in proper perspective" (Mangold, 1980, p. 96).

Classmates generally perceived the student with a visual impairment to be incapable of participation in many of their activities. This was frequently reported to be justification for classmates to exclude the child with a visual impairment from their play, as evidenced in the following excerpt:

I: *Tell me how kids in your class feel about playing outside at recess or noon hour with Tony (child who is blind).*

R: *Well sometime, most of the time, we try and get away from him because he can't do much that we can do, like run, because he'll get lost and run into people and stuff. So either we walk around with him and stuff or, or he's with a teacher walking.*

I: *Is it easier or more difficult for him to make friends than other kids in your class?*

R: *Ah...it's pretty difficult for him to make friends because lots of people don't like him.*

I: *Tell me about that.*

R: *Well, because he can't do as many things as they can. Yeah, that's why cuz they wanta do this but he can't do that so they just kinda don't play with him. [Grade 3]*

Since being able to do what others were doing was critical to participation, classmates' perceptions that the student with a visual impairment could not do many of the things they did was a significant deterrent to being sought out as a "best friend."

Even when the child with a visual impairment appeared to be participating with relative ease in most playground activities, peers perceived themselves as having to make an extra effort if they were to include the visually impaired child in their play:

I: *Tell me how kids in your class feel about playing outside at recess or noon hour with Lisa.*
R: *Well, they feel quite hard to, to play and that because when they're playing something or playing a game it's hard for her to understand and see the way your pointing or what, what you're showing is the base and that, and who's "it." [Grade 1]*

The perception that being a friend to a student with a visual impairment required extra effort appeared to become more evident with the increasing age of the children and the advancement of skill level necessary for active participation in typical playground activities. The convictions children held related to the inability of a child with a visual impairment to do what other children were doing frequently seemed obscured by the practical concerns associated with the extra effort entailed if this child was to be included.

In the classroom the child with a visual impairment was generally perceived to be able to do what the other children were doing but the slower working rate and the large, often "messy-looking" appearance of the handwork of the child with a visual impairment seemed to be interpreted as evidence of incompetence or a lower level of ability. In addition, it became apparent during the interviews that although children perceived adaptive materials as necessary or helpful for their classmate with a visual impairment, use of such materials seemed to prejudice the perception children who were sighted constructed in relation to the quality of performance of the student. The following excerpt is typical of the responses classmates made in relation to the school performance of students who were visually impaired:

I: *Tell me how kids in your class feel about working in school with Lisa (student with a visual impairment) .*
R: *Not really good.*
I: *No. Can you tell me about that?*
R: *Cuz she doesn't do the proper stuff, like, em, she can't read too good, and everybody's just, and ah, so if you're her partner then ah, they would just say, "Lisa, we're on the first page," and, and she's only on the first page and I'm on the second page. Or stay like that until class is over cuz Lisa'll say, "What's this word?" when you read and she only reads the easy words. [Grade 1]*

In this excerpt the classmate's reference to the "proper stuff" was associated with the student's use of large print as opposed to regular print texts. By using the large print text and not the ones used by other members of the class, the child with a visual impairment was perceived as not doing what everyone else was doing. Since the level of difficulty of reading materials in elementary grades is generally directly proportional to the print size used, the larger print used by students with a visual impairment was perceived to be "easier work" than that of classmates, when in fact, the reading material was identical. This finding was noted at all four sites where students with low vision were print readers.

There was also the perception that work completed using adaptive materials or equipment was of lesser quality than that produced through regular means (e.g., work written on dark-lined paper was perceived to look less attractive than that completed on regular-lined paper). In addition, at the upper elementary levels, classmates were beginning to consider the use of such equipment by their classmate with a visual impairment as providing an unfair advantage to the student, as can be seen in the following typical responses to the question, "What do kids your age think about him using these special things in class?"

[Excerpt 1]

R: *I think he's pretty lucky. Because it's easier to read the books and I'd get done faster if I had one of those [referring to large print text]. [Grade 6]*

[Excerpt 2]

R: *They think, I think that they say, "That's not fair!" or "Why does he get to use that and I don't get to do that?" [referring to unlimited use of a computer to complete written assignments]. [Grade 5]*

Classmates who reported the use of special materials by the child with a visual impairment did not bother them or those who were pleased it was of help to the student, tended to be above average students who consistently performed at a higher level than the student who was visually impaired. Interestingly, those students who were at similar academic levels as the student with a visual impairment, particularly in a competitive environment, seemed to be the ones most threatened by the child's use of adaptive aids.

Pupil Assumption 3: *To be part of a group a child ought to initiate interaction with others in the group to gain access to the group.*

On school playgrounds, children frequently gather as a group to participate in a variety of activities (e.g., skipping, marbles, play fighting). Those who are not "best friends" with a participant or not one of the initial organizers of the activity must gain access to the group in specific ways. They may ask the person who started the game, ask the person who brought the ball, or ask someone they know in the group to promote their admission to the group among the other participants. Such groups rarely seek members and children who wait to be invited to participate in playground activities are invariably left out.

The act of initiating interaction with peers was frequently problematic for all of the students who were visually impaired. Although three of these children seemed to possess particularly good conversational skills and were considered to be extroverts by their teachers, they often appeared awkward and visibly uncomfortable in their attempts to initiate conversation or join groups with classmates. They tended to go from group to group on the playground and participate in random activities, as opposed to consistently interacting with a particular classmate or group of children.

For the student in the study who was totally blind, initiating interaction presented some unique situations. For example, one day after approximately a month and a half of school, the student was asked whom he wanted for a partner for a particular activity. He responded, "I don't know. I don't even know who's in this class." In a large class, quiet children may be almost unknown to a classmate who is blind. Further investigation of this type of predicament revealed rather startling findings. Often on the playground, this boy was not even aware of the names of the children with whom he was playing. Everyday he tended to participate in the same activity, in the same location, throughout the duration of the recess. Other children tended to change activities more frequently and hence, participants in his activity were not constant. When asked how he chose a playmate, he replied, "I don't. They choose." In the confusion and activity involving over 350 students on a playground, this boy could not seek out playmates he desired or even changes in activities. He was restricted to those children who chose to initiate contact with him. Undoubtedly, children with severe vision loss (i.e., not totally blind but severely visually impaired) experience comparable difficulties.

Similarly, in class, students with a visual impairment initiated interaction less frequently and appeared to be constrained in a number of other ways. First, because they had very slow reading and writing rates, they rarely finished an assignment in time to interact with classmates who had completed the task and were socializing between activities. Second, these students seemed better able to capture the attention of the teacher than the attention of a classmate. For the most part, even when amidst their classmates, the student with a visual impairment routinely sought out the teacher with whom to initiate and participate in conversation rather than a classmate.

Interestingly, the classmates of the student with a visual impairment perceived this child as making little effort to join in, disinterested in doing what the others were doing, or behaving inappropriately when attempting to join a group. The following excerpt is an example of one student's "entry behaviour" and the reaction of silence generated by his approach:

> [Recess is being held inside because it is raining.] Tony (student who is blind) returns to the classroom about 5 minutes late with a very pleased expression on his face and announces, "I made it by myself." He puts his cane in the corner and says to himself, "Cane up," and then jumps excitedly. He goes over to the boys playing with the blocks. Daniel,

> Matthew, and Colin are building a tower together while Adam and Tyler are working on individual construction. Tony says, "What are you doing? Are you allowed playing with the blocks? I want to play too." The boys ignore these questions and Tyler lets him take some blocks from his pile as he sits on the floor near the others. Tony picks up two blocks and bangs them together and then bangs one on the palm of his hand and rocks a bit. No one is paying any attention to him and he says, "You know what you should do?" No response. He continues, "Put blocks under your houses you're making." No response. "What are you making?" Daniel replies, "A tower." Tony asks, "Can I help?" Matthew replies, "Not yet, Tony, not yet." Tony sits with his head down resting on his knee and pressing his eye. Then he takes a few blocks and says, "I know what I'm going to make." Trevor who has just arrived says, "What, Tony?" Tony says, "You guys pretend there's a bridge going up to the tower. Pretend there's a draw bridge." The boys building the tower do not respond. Tony repeats his suggestion but the boys don't answer. Tony says, "I'll build a draw bridge, okay?" No answer. "You guys want a draw bridge?" Tyler replies, "We're not building a castle we're building a tower." Their tower keeps falling as they try to increase the height. They say to Trevor who comes near, "Don't make it fall down!" Tony sits and bangs on his palm with a block. Then Tony says, "You guys, I'm building a draw bridge up to the tower." The boys don't answer and Tyler and Adam who have now started individual projects, begin to argue over the blocks. Trevor goes over to Adam and accuses him of taking all the blocks. The bell rings and Tony immediately starts to help them pick up the blocks. [Observation notes]

In this excerpt, Tony's classmates effectively exclude him from their activity, although he is permitted to participate in a similar activity on the fringe of the group because classroom rules would dictate such. Tony's lack of competence in making the rather elaborate constructions of his classmates may also have contributed to their actions to deny him access to their group. However, Tony's "entry behaviour" was contrary to that generally condoned by the pupil culture. Children who successfully join groups initially stand back and observe; when the time is right, ask permission to join; and continue to participate in the same activity as the other children. Those who experience difficulty joining groups tend to try to dominate the group, act aggressively, and attempt to change the original form of play in which the group was involved. What becomes obvious in analyzing the excerpt involving Tony is that it is impossible for one who is blind to comply with some of the behaviours other students believe to be appropriate when joining groups (e.g., observe the action of the group before asking to join). Research findings have suggested that joining an existing group or activity may be one of the more complex social skills children, in general, have to learn (Corsaro, 1981; Gottman & Parker, 1986).

Children with a visual impairment who were perceived by peers to behave inappropriately when attempting to join their groups were generally reported to behave in ways characteristic of those experiencing difficulty joining groups. That is, they "barged in" without asking, were "bossy," or wouldn't "let you do what you want to do." However, due to loss of vision, it was impossible for Tony to stay at the fringe of the activity and observe the activities of the participants of the group before attempting to join. Considering the reluctance of the boys to provide him with the information he requested, that is, information children who were fully sighted would have access to through observation, Tony had few alternatives but to "barge in" and to be assertive in accessing the information he needed to know to participate effectively. Unfortunately, in doing so, he alienated himself from the group.

A second type of behaviour frequently observed in students with a visual impairment was a "hovering type" of manoeuvre. They would stand on the fringe of a group, apparently waiting to be included but not initiating any action to join. In fact, without classmates understanding the predicament faced by the student with a visual impairment, it is unlikely these students could learn to routinely join groups involved in certain types of activities. Entry to many groups requires visual skills and access to visual information which is just not available to the student with a severe vision loss. Therefore, in general, on the playground students with a visual impairment could best be described as "on the fringe" of interaction with their peers. From the perspective of classmates, these students had acquired a reputation of not behaving appropriately or not wanting to do anything.

Pupil Assumption 4: Boys and girls ought not to be "best friends."

In the early years of elementary school boys and girls can often be seen playing together in groups. Despite the less exclusive groups characteristic of this age, boys and girls still have only same gender "best friends" during school hours. In the upper elementary grades, groups become increasingly exclusive both by gender and popularity. When a boy and girl routinely associate with one another on the playground, they are considered to be romantically involved. A more common interaction between upper elementary boys and girls on the playground is "bugging," a form of teasing initiated by either a boy or girl with a member of the opposite sex. "Bugging" can be a good-natured game enjoyed among friends with much laughter and playfulness or one centred upon children who are mocked or tormented by the majority of children on the playground.

Interestingly, in this study three of the four boys with a visual impairment routinely interacted with girls, both in the classroom and on the playground. Because they were aware of the accepted cultural norm, that is, boys don't play with girls, interaction with girls sometimes created a dilemma for them, as can be seen in the following discussion with a grade five boy with a visual impairment:

I: *Which kids would you choose to work with on a class project?*
R: *Lee, David, Kevin, Daniel, and Colin.*
I: *Tell me about them.*
R: *They're all good at working at projects and things.*
I: *Which kids would you not choose to work with on a project in class?*
R: *Hmm. Marla, Lisa, Matthew, Ashley, Ryan, Wendell, Jacklyn..Donna, Darren, Morgan, Michelle, Jodi, or Dana, or Aleasha. [Rhymes them off.]*
I: *Tell me about them.*
R: *Well, half, half them are stupid at working on projects, and a couple of them are pretty good but I don't want to work with girls.*
I: *Oh, tell me about that.*
R: *About what?*
I: *Not wanting to work with girls.*
R: *Because, oh, it gives me the shivers, I hate working with girls. They bug me.*
I: *Now, I'm a little bit confused here because you, your group is all girls [he sits in a classroom group with four girls].*
R: *Oh, yeah. Yes, that's cuz they always, they want me to. [They want him to sit with their group.]*
I: *Oh, okay. You haven't moved your seat up beside, let's see, Lee, or..*
R: *No, I know they don't want me to, really.*
I: *Oh, I see.*
R: *They're happy in their groups.*
I: *Tell me about the seating arrangement in your class? I find it very interesting.*
R: *Cuz at first I was at the counter, where the pencil sharpener was, with four other people, then I moved over by, by myself, then I moved with Darren and Matthew [the two most unpopular boys in the class], then I moved by myself again for a few days, and then I moved back with, over there to Dana [four girls sitting in a group who allowed him to join them] and them. The reason I sit there is so Jodi and them can help me sometimes, cuz I can't read some of the prints.*
I: *Oh, okay. And why wouldn't you sit with Daniel and David [boys he earlier named as "best friends"]?*
R: *I would, I would if they'd let me.*
I: *Oh, they won't let you.*
R: *Like they, it's not that they don't like me, it's just that they have a group of four already [there were no limits placed on the group size] and they wouldn't want, and they don't really want me to sit there.*

Whether through past experience or other interactions, this boy perceived children of the same gender to be his appropriate play or workmates. However, he also perceived them to be inaccessible to him and chose girls who "gave him the shivers" as one alternative to being alone.

This acceptance and inclusion of boys who were visually impaired by female classmates and the routine exclusion of male students with a visual impairment by their male classmates was noted throughout the study. When children had to choose partners, most often the student with a visual impairment was the last or among the last chosen. Their partners were, in most cases, girls. Both on the playground and in the classroom the boys who were visually impaired interacted predominately with girls. As well, girls more frequently volunteered to help or work with their classmate who was visually impaired. Thus, the types of relationships and activities observed for boys with a visual impairment and their female classmates were different than those for boys who were fully sighted. This frequently resulted in the boys who were visually impaired being isolated from interaction with other male classmates.

Spender (1982, p. 85) stated that girls act as a "negative reference group, against which boys' performance is enhanced." In this study it appeared that male students with a visual impairment were devalued among their male peers (i.e., not often viewed as acceptable workmates or playmates), but were more acceptable to girls who, in general, tend to serve as the negative reference group for boys under usual circumstances. The nurturing role to which girls are socialized in our society may also have been reflected in their greater tendency to interact with and accept their male classmates who were visually impaired. However, if students with a visual impairment become increasingly isolated from their same-gender peer group as they proceed through elementary school, as seemed to be indicated in this study and that of both Eaglestein (1975) and Goupil and Comeau (1983), girls who are visually impaired may be at a greater risk socially than are boys who are visually impaired. Boys would conceivably still have the more accepting female group of classmates upon which to draw for companionship, even if just during classroom hours.

The complexity of the situation and the vulnerability of the boys who were visually impaired was further evidenced when the perceptions of the classmates of these boys were examined. The tendency of boys who were visually impaired to associate primarily with girls was considered inappropriate by the majority of their male peers but not so by their female peers. Those male classmates who expressed opposition to the camaraderie between their male classmate with a visual impairment and female members of the class seemed unable to comprehend why this boy would choose to associate with girls even when they themselves, openly reported a preference not to play or work with him. In short, boys with a visual impairment were perceived to have chosen females rather than male associates despite the less than receptive behaviour routinely exhibited toward them by their male classmates:

I: *You mentioned you wouldn't want Jamie [student with a visual impairment] to sit at your table.*

R: *He likes sitting with girls. Even on the playground, cuz that's where you always see him..with girls. [Grade 5]*

Obviously, the students with a visual impairment were in a precarious position with regard to boy-girl relationships. The more accepting attitude of girls and the ability of the student who was visually impaired to better participate in the generally less physically challenging activities of girls (e.g., swinging, talking in groups, playing house), provided more opportunities for meaningful interaction than did activities with boys. From the perspective of their male classmates, boys who played with girls were "wimps" and were, therefore, not desirable playmates. Thus, boy-girl relationships condoned by the pupil culture created an impasse for male students with a visual impairment. For them, it was a "Catch-22" situation.

Pupil Assumption 5: *Unpopular children ought to play with other unpopular children.*

It was disheartening to observe the isolation and the struggles of unpopular children in the elementary schools in this study. They were blatantly excluded from group activities both on the playground and, where possible, in the classroom. Although most did not become "best friends" with another unpopular child, they associated with this child as an alternative to being alone. Rejected children, those who were not accepted by most children in the school, were most often seen in proximity to rejected children from other classes.

In this study, none of the children with a visual impairment were members of an identified "popular gang" or played with such children on the playground. They seemed to possess somewhat of a neutral position in relation to popularity. They were not sought out by classmates, as were popular children, nor were they the brunt of significant amounts of teasing or of physical tormenting, as were many unpopular children. When classmates were asked how they chose a partner for an activity, they consistently reported selecting their "best friends." However, students with a visual impairment did not appear to perceive the same option available to them. Whether their visual limitations made it impossible to act quickly enough to locate a partner, either by calling out their name or through non-verbal gestures, or whether other children avoided them, it was evident they were most frequently partners with less popular children.

In the following two excerpts, Peter, one boy with a visual impairment, and a female classmate, Allison, are responding to the interviewer's questions about how one goes about getting a partner for an activity:

I: *Peter, when you have a partner in gym you usually have Paula, Allison, or Cathy.*
R: *Yeah.*
I: *You don't have David or Nathan.*
R: *Cuz they're always with someone else. See we're allowed to choose, they choose their own partners. I just take who ever is left.*
I: *Oh, I see. Is that how you do it in the class?*
R: *Yes, that's the only thing that works. [Grade 4]*

It would seem that the consideration of prime importance for the student who is visually impaired is just getting a partner. Allison, Peter's classmate who is fully sighted , seems to perceive this situation similarly:

I: *Allison, how do you go about getting a partner when the teacher tells you to get a partner for an activity?*

R: *Oh, you pick one of your friends that somebody else hasn't picked. I always go for the girls and sometimes if Cathy's [girl rejected by classmates] the only one left, usually, sometimes if there's, if she's the only one left I go with Peter.*

Situations necessitating the choosing of partners by classmates seemed to place the student with a visual impairment at risk because they were rarely chosen until the end. These students perceived themselves to have little choice in the selection of a partner, but rather to be destined to "take who's ever left." For the most part, classmates of these students held similar perceptions.

Pupil Assumption 6: *Children ought not associate with unpopular children.*

Within pupil culture, association with unpopular children, for purposes other than teasing or mistreating them, detracts from a student's popularity. Even being assigned by the teacher as a partner to an unpopular child is considered bad for one's reputation. Students can also harm their reputation and, thus chances for developing friendships, by associating or having a reputation of associating with "bad" or "weird" people during after school hours.

Unpopular children are judged more harshly by their classmates than are popular children. In this study, classmates routinely underestimated the level of performance of their less popular peers in areas such as skill level in the gym, contributions to discussions, and quality of work. Popular children, on the other hand, appeared to enjoy a much higher level of tolerance relative to both performance and behaviour. They were either judged less critically by peers or they were forgiven their weaknesses.

For children with a visual impairment, the choice of partners or a playmate often seemed more related to who was physically close at hand, who happened to be participating in the limited activities enjoyed by the student, or who was willing to accommodate the child with a visual impairment in a particular game. However, given the exclusion of less popular children by their popular classmates, the chances that a child with a visual impairment would interact with an unpopular child were greater. In the classroom where all children were more accessible to students with a visual impairment, they interacted more frequently with a range of children. However, when partners were chosen, they were often left to be with the unpopular classmates.

The two younger children with visual impairments in this study appeared to experience some difficulties in relation to their perceptions of who was popular and unpopular. A similar misinterpretation in their perceptions of their popularity in relation to their classmates was also noted. However, the three upper elementary boys seemed to identify the same children as unpopular as did their sighted peers and to make choices about their interaction with these peers. The grade six boy who was visually impaired had a "best friend" who was rejected by the other children in the classroom. He perceived his "best friend" as unpopular and also seemed to be aware that he was in the same category as his friend. Yet, for students who were visually impaired, being without anybody was not a pleasant alternative.

Pupil Assumption 7: ***To be part of the class, children ought to like the same things as their classmates, dress the same as their classmates, and act the same as their classmates.***

In our society, there is tremendous pressure for children to be alike. In the schools observed in this study, children aspired to be like their classmates. To be different was to invite hostility or rejection from classmates. Nonconformity, whether in dress or behaviour was openly reprimanded by classmates. Furthermore, considerable effort to dress and act like a "best friend" was frequently a prerequisite to acceptance.

The children with a visual impairment in this study did not usually dress differently than the majority of their classmates. Charles, the boy in Grade 6, was somewhat overprotected by his mother and would arrive in school wearing snowpants. This practice was shunned by classmates who viewed the wearing of snowpants as "babyish." As children proceed through elementary school they become more assertive in their choice of clothing and a parent's taste in fashion is usually met with disapproval. Within pupil culture, there is a "uniform" appropriate to any given age group (e.g., T-shirts and jogging pants, blue jeans and sweaters). Parents of children with a visual impairment must be alert to the styles dictated by pupil culture and sensitive to the implications conformity has in relation to their child's social acceptance by peers. Inappropriate dress does not necessarily lead to rejection by classmates but frequently discourages children from initiating interaction or associating with a child who does not adhere to the dress code of the group. Unlike dress, "act the same as their classmates" is an aspect of pupil culture which cannot be easily interpreted. Actions or behaviour are not components which can be independently examined in isolation from the process of interaction. According to Fine (1981), actions or behaviours are subjected to different levels of tolerance depending upon the nature of the relationship in which one is interacting. In the presence of good friends one's actions are judged less harshly than when interacting with those who are merely acquaintances.

For the students who were visually impaired, there were actions and behaviours which deviated from what might be considered conventional everyday behaviours of children who were fully sighted. These differences can be categorized in two ways. First, there were those associated with a visual impairment, such as involuntary eye movement, close working distance when reading and writing, or difficulties associated with free and independent mobility within the school environment. Second, and more difficult to describe, there was an awkwardness experienced in interactions between a child who was visually impaired and a classmate which was not evident in similar exchanges between two or more classmates who were fully sighted. It seemed the children had not been able to resolve the aspects of interaction stress which prevented them from developing real friendships with a student with a visual impairment. That is, the spontaneous acceptance of children with disabilities anticipated by advocates of integration had not seemed to have evolved.

All of the children who were visually impaired perceived themselves to be different from their peers because they had a visual impairment. They reported, "We can't do as many things as other kids." They also perceived their visual impairment to hinder the process of making friends and to be the subject of teasing by classmates. Although the boys in this study did not believe they were distinguishable from their peers by appearance, the child with albinism did perceive herself to be different in appearance. She complained of being teased by older children on the playground. This teasing seemed to centre more upon her appearance than her visual impairment. Vander Kolk and Bright (1983), in their research on albinism, concluded that the albino's "extraordinary physical features tend to have a stronger impact on others than the limited vision" (p. 49). Although it was not apparent whether this child perceived her appearance to be more responsible for her being different from peers than her visual impairment, she did, indeed, perceive herself to be different.

Perceptions of differences in relation to their behaviour were almost nonexistent among the children with a visual impairment. Even those with obvious mannerisms did not perceive their actions as different from those of their peers. The child who was totally blind, in particular, was unaware of the reaction of children to his constant bouncing, particularly when he was standing beside them and in physical contact with them. He was aware it annoyed them but not of how "different" others perceived him to be. He even did it purposefully to tease. However, he was not aware that children purposefully avoided getting near him in the lineups, exchanged glances of disgust or annoyance when he jumped about, or ran from him when he called for them as he was standing bouncing in one spot. Although he complained that "kids" in his class wouldn't play with him on the playground, he did not seem cognizant of the possible association with his atypical behaviour.

In some respects, this child's lack of knowledge about how his behaviour was interpreted by others is similar to the restrictions on information children with visual impairments receive in relation to comparing their competence to that of their peers. They must rely on those in their environment to give them accurate messages about how their behaviour is perceived by others since their access to such information is limited. Without feedback relevant to their inappropriate actions, they could not conform to the criteria for acceptance inherent to many aspects of pupil culture.

It was difficult to ascertain the extent to which the peers of these students perceived them to act differently than other children. During observation, it was not uncommon to notice classmates laugh, roll their eyes, stare, or exchange glances of annoyance or disgust in response to the behaviour of the student with a visual impairment. Yet, in interviews these peers tended to emphasize the fact that the child was "blind" rather than focus on the specific idiosyncrasies of her/his behaviour. Once again it appeared as if different behaviour or expectations for different behaviour were inherent to the state of being "visually impaired." Following is an excerpt from one of the few interviews with a classmate in which the different behaviour of the student who was visually impaired was elaborated upon by a peer:

I: *What's it like being Peter's [student with a visual impairment] partner in the gym?*

R: *Oh, well, if we're just practising for floor hockey, not floor hockey but, um volleyball, something like volleyball.. but he can't, like ah, he can't usually get it over the net.*

I: *Umhmm. So what's it like being his partner?*

R: *Well, I try to get somebody that can throw it, like, cuz that get it's done, gets it done faster.*

I: *Peter gets good marks in school. What do you think about this?*

R: *Yeah, sometimes he gets good marks like, on his tests. But he's still not in the popular group.*

I: *You said he has trouble seeing. How is his behaviour different from other children?*

R: *Ah, oh, well, like, when he gets excited sometimes he squeals. Like he makes a noise and that means, like, he's real excited and he moves his arms [motions arm flapping]. Like when he, when he's talking he moves his arms back and forth and his eyes are all moving everywhere, when, when he's not, even if he's just doing his work his eyes sometimes go over here and over here. They don't usually stay in one place.*

I: *You mentioned that his eyes move around and when he's talking to you he doesn't look at you. What do you think about that?*

R: *Well-l-l, he doesn't, he looks at me like. But like, when we're talking, like, he looks at me and sometimes he moves his head when he's talking, like. Well, he just does that cuz he's part blind and he, he, he's different from other children.*

I: *What makes him different from other children?*

R: *Oh, because he's blind, like he's half blind and he can't do his things, like, he can't do the same things as other children can.*

I: *How does it make you feel when his eyes move around like that?*

R: *Ohh, I got use to it when, he was in my class for a coup.., a lot of years, maybe three or four or so. And, he was my friend, like sometimes I liked to play with him when I had nobody else. [Grade 4]*

Even though few classmates spontaneously reported the child with a visual impairment to act differently than other children in the class, when asked specifically about "different behaviour" of these children, responses centred upon the mannerisms typically associated with children with a visual impairment. Things such as arm flapping or jumping about when excited, not making eye contact, or standing too close when speaking with someone were often mentioned. For the most part, classmates of students with a visual impairment perceived these different behaviours to be undesirable.

Pupil Assumption 8: ***"Best friends" ought to help each other in noncompetitive situations as well as in competitive situations when they are on the same team.***

With class sizes in this study as large as 28 children, it was often difficult for the teacher to provide the level of assistance students required when it was needed. Therefore, students routinely relied on assistance from classmates to enable them to complete their work. Children with one or more "best friends" in the class were at a definite advantage in soliciting help from classmates. Those without friends or with only "okay friends" frequently had requests for assistance ignored or denied. "Best friends" rarely rejected requests for help unless the two friends were on opposite teams or were competing for academic standing in the class.

In comparison to their peers who were sighted, two of the children with a visual impairment in this study received an inordinate amount of help from both classmates and teachers; one received more help than the majority of peers and the other two approximately the same amount as their peers. However, the relationship between "best friends" and willingness to help was different for the children with a visual impairment than it was for their classmates. It appeared that a classmate need not be a "best friend" of the student who was visually impaired in order to volunteer to help. Furthermore, classmates rarely refused to help when assistance was requested by the student with a visual impairment. Such was not always the case if the student did not have a disability.

Two other aspects of the helping relationship between children with a visual impairment and their peers were prominent. First, the opportunities for the children with a visual impairment to reciprocate the help they received were limited. Although all were willing to help, situational circumstances (e.g., the extended time required to finish a task) and other contextual factors (e.g., capability of detecting those in need of help) resulted in infrequent reciprocation of assistance they routinely received from peers. Second, the students with a visual impairment seldom verbally thanked those who helped them. From an observer's point of view, it seemed as if such help was an indistinguishable aspect of the situation, that is, taken for granted by the students with a visual impairment. From the perspective of these students, the necessity for assistance seemed to be inseparable from some activities and, therefore, not perceived as "help" but merely as a component of the activity.

The main contention of this eighth assumption is that it is primarily the role of "best friends" to help one another. However, perceptions related to this criteria for friendship were different for the five children with a visual impairment in this study. For the most part, a peer would help but would not necessarily continue the interaction once the help had been provided. As well, the teacher was observed to be the main source of assistance both in the classroom and on the playground.

The child who was totally blind in this study believed he needed help with many more things than did those who had low vision. Even those things he was capable of doing independently, he interpreted as situations in which peers could continue to assist him. However, he did not understand the connection between "best friend" relationships and helping. Most peers were expected to help. There was also a sense that his perception of helping was more like the concept of companionship than helping. His understanding of the help he received from the teacher assistant also seemed to indicate a different perception of helping:

I: *This year Mrs. Matheson [teacher assistant] goes with you to gym. Last year she didn't. Tell me about this.*
R: *[pause] I don't know, well, she's pretty nice, to take, to help me in gym.*
I: *So last year she didn't help you and this year she does. Can you tell me why it's different this year?*
R: *I don't know. You'd have to ask her. I don't know. I never asked her.*
I: *What do you think?*
R: *Ah, I don't know, like, I think she likes helping me. [Grade 3]*

There seemed to be a sense that others enjoyed helping him and he, in turn, both appreciated the help which made the completion of many tasks less cumbersome. As well, he was delighted by interaction with his peers.

Common to all 31 classmates interviewed at the five different sites (i.e., the five to eight classmates of each student with a visual impairment), was the perception that the student with a visual impairment required a substantial amount of help and although they were not "best friends" with this student, they were obligated or at least expected to routinely assist. Despite evidence from observation that only two of the children with a visual impairment actually received an inordinate amount of help from their peers, all those interviewed reported providing assistance to the student with a visual impairment.

Interestingly, it appeared that most interaction with the student with a visual impairment, whether involving assistance or not, was perceived to entail assistance. Even when the student with a visual impairment was paired with a less capable student for a particular activity and completed the major part of the assignment, the classmate perceived this situation as one in which he/she had been helping the student who was visually impaired.

Pupil Assumption 9: *Children ought to play with children from their own classroom.*

As mentioned earlier in the text, at the beginning of the school year there appear to be loosely defined play groups. Children from various classes intermingle on a limited basis. As the school year proceeds, classroom friends become "best friends" and the class itself becomes an exclusive group. Students who play with children from classes other than their own tend to be those who are rejected by their classmates and who must seek companionship among less popular children from other classes. Even children who are "best friends" during out-of-school hours choose to play with classmates rather than their out-of-school friends during school hours.

In comparison to their peers who were fully sighted, children with a visual impairment spent much less time with their own classmates on the playground. Instead, they were frequently observed playing with children from other classes and even children from the younger grades. All of the children with a visual impairment expressed a yearning to play with those classmates they perceived as popular although none routinely interacted with these popular classmates on the playground. As is evident in the following excerpt, students who were visually impaired perceived themselves to have limited control and little choice with respect to whom they could play:

I: *When I asked you earlier about what kids [classmates] do on the playground, you said you didn't know what the kids did?*
R: *Yeah. They probably, they play soccer. Some of them.*
I: *Umhmm. Know anything else that they do out there?*
R: *Play tag...like most of the people, I ask to play with them, "Oh, no, I'm playing with someone else." So, like, I don't usually play with them, I just, like I have to walk around by myself. It's hard.*
[Later in the interview]
I: *Who are the kids in your class that the other kids do not seem to play with very often?*
R: *I don't know, because, like, I don't hang around with them. I don't hang around much with no kids in my class. [Grade 3]*

Peers of the student with a visual impairment, despite their reluctance to play with this student, did not condone the tendency of this student to play with those who were not classmates. However, the regular association of one of the students who was visually impaired with a playmate from a lower grade was frowned upon by his classmates and perceived as being a significant difference in behaviour when compared to other children:

I: *You said he was different than most kids?*
R: *Well, he can't see good and he uses a typewriter in class, everything, so.*
I: *How about in the way he acts?*
R: *Well, in the way he acts, he only likes to play with the grade fours, no one older or his age or something. [Grade 5]*

Therefore, similar to the situation which developed in relation to boy-girl relationships, when students with a visual impairment sought companionship outside the sanctioned boundaries for interaction, they were perceived to be behaving inappropriately. It also appeared that the more capable or competent a student with a visual impairment was perceived to be, the more harshly he/she was judged when his/her behaviour was discerned to be inappropriate.

Pupil Assumption 10: *Children ought to follow the rules negotiated within the school culture.*

As in all cultures, pupil culture is characterized by rules which have evolved in relation to the needs of its members. In this study, rules varied somewhat from school to school but at all sites children were often reprimanded or ostracized by others when they did not follow the rules. In the classroom, rules made by the teacher (e.g., "Stay in your seat while I'm doing the demonstration." or "Don't count on your fingers.") which were not adhered to, would bring reprimands from classmates, particularly if the offender was an unpopular child. There were also rules made by the children, such as, "You can help another student but don't let them copy your work." or "Don't tell the substitute teacher about extra work which was supposed to be handed in that day." On the playground where children were more in control, they had rules related to play such as, "You can't join in the game without asking," or "When you say you'll play with someone you can't just walk away and leave them."

Students with a visual impairment tended to follow the rules when they were aware of them. However, some rules were more difficult for children with a visual impairment to ascertain than others. For example, how to act when talking with a classmate of a different gender or how cooperative to be with teachers seemed to be particularly troublesome for the students with a visual impairment. These types of exchanges tended to be characterized by subtle rules negotiated between teachers and pupils during the everyday interactions in the classroom (e.g., how much information to provide in response to a question, the distinction between "goody-goody" and acceptable behaviour). Children with a visual impairment were at risk on several levels in such interactions. First, they had difficulty interpreting the subtle messages essential to incorporate the necessary information into appropriate behaviour. Second, when they did respond inappropriately, particularly in the classroom, they did not see the reactions of their classmates. Expressions of disgust or annoyance, exchanged glances of ridicule and/or humour, or the rolling of eyes went unnoticed. Third, peers seemed reluctant to verbally reprimand children with a visual impairment when they behaved inappropriately, especially if in proximity to a teacher.

In attempting to assist a child with a visual impairment, teachers sometimes inadvertently encouraged her/him to disobey rules of the pupil culture. For example, by asking students to play during recess with their classmate who was visually impaired, teachers helped the student with a visual impairment gain access to a group or interfere in a "best friend" relationship in ways which ignored conventional rules of access applicable to other pupils. A similar problem occurred in the classroom when the teacher unconsciously or with good intentions provided assistance, which was not available to classmates, to the student with the visual impairment. Thus, when students with a visual impairment did not receive the necessary information and feedback to enhance socialization into the existing pupil culture or when teachers interfered in ways which were incompatible with negotiated rules of pupil culture, the social acceptance of students with a visual impairment was placed at risk.

Although the children who were visually impaired believed they usually followed the rules, they also had a sense of having a degree of immunity because they were visually impaired. They perceived themselves as being "special" in relation to their classmates and as receiving special treatment from teachers:

I: *What do the kids in your class think about you always being at the front of the line to go to French?*
R: *I don't know. I think they think it's pretty..bad, like, I think, I think they feel kinda left out. I don't know why..why they would.*
I: *Why do you think they might?*
R: *Maybe they think that they're, well, I know there are some people that don't think I'm very special. I know I'm not, but I mean...but the teacher treats me like I'm very special.*
I: *Umhmm. Which teachers?*
R: *Most all, mostly all of them. [Grade 3]*

Students with a visual impairment seemed to distinguish "special privileges" in school as inherent to being visually impaired.

When children with a visual impairment did not follow the rules on the playground, the consequences were similar to those for most children, that is, rejection or reprimand by their peers. However, these consequences were frequently not as harsh for students with a visual impairment as they were for other nonconforming students. Although classmates could identify situations in which the student with a visual impairment did not conform, they tended to be perplexed about how to deal with such behaviour in the classroom situation. Classmates perceived it to be "risky to straighten out" a student with a visual impairment in the presence of teachers.

The peers of students with a visual impairment perceived these children to be treated differently by their teachers. Following are excerpts from four different schools which illustrate classmates' perception that students with a visual impairment are granted privileges or treatment not accorded the general student body:

[Excerpt 1]
R: *Like Peter, they, he [the teacher] has to give extra attention to him cuz like, when we win prizes usually nobody pays any attention but whenever he wins prizes everybody in the class, even the teacher's going around saying, "You're doing good, Peter. That's excellent," and all*

that and he gets really excited about it cuz, like they're trying to be as nice as they can to him.

I: *Does he get more attention than other kids?*

R: *Well, sometimes cuz he's blind and he needs more help. [Grade 4]*

[Excerpt 2]

I: *And you were telling me he doesn't see so good?*

R: *Yeah.*

I: *Tell me about people who don't see so good.*

R: *Um, well sometimes the teachers treat them a little better.*

I: *A little better?*

R: *Yeah. But I didn't find that very fair that Kevin [a classmate] got taken off the computer, just so he [the student with a visual impairment] could do something there.*

I: *Umhmm.*

R: *It's not fair. [Grade 5]*

[Excerpt 3]

R: *Sometimes the teacher, ah, lets him go for a drink or somewhere like that and she doesn't let the rest of the class go. Then ah, that might make the other people feel insulted because he gets special attention. [Grade 3]*

[Excerpt 4]

R: *Well, she gets more help than us. That's what we're kinda jealous about. Lots of people. [Grade 1]*

Because of the perceived special treatment of students with a visual impairment by their teachers, it was difficult to ascertain whether classmates faulted the student for not following rules or if their perception of injustice was primarily associated with the teacher's treatment of this child. Given the facial expressions of annoyance and exchanged glances of resentment, this perception of injustice did not appear to enhance this child's acceptance by peers.

Pupil Assumption 11: *Friends ought to reciprocate the actions of their friends, whether positive or negative.*

Davies (1982) reported that when "best friends" interact they respond often in seemingly direct imitation to one another's behaviour. A similar phenomena was noted in this study. If one child complimented another on her/his art work, the child receiving the compliment made a similarly positive comment about the friend's art work. If a friend became suddenly uncooperative or "mouthy," this behaviour was reciprocated. This pattern of reciprocity among children was most prominent during exchanges of physical contact where children could frequently be heard to comment about the need to "pay back" a classmate for some action, predominately a negative one.

In the classroom it was also observed that reciprocity was all important. Classmates who were chosen as desirable partners for projects or assignments were those who would do "their fair share" or who would not "just sit and let you do all the work." When children worked in groups and one child received assistance from another, the recipient could often be seen to volunteer some form of unsolicited advice or assistance in reciprocation.

Some of the difficulties children with a visual impairment encountered in reciprocating assistance received from their peers were mentioned earlier in relation to the cultural assumption that "best friends" help. In addition, for classmates, negative reciprocation proved troublesome when it involved the child with a visual impairment. When posing interview questions involving a scenario in which the child with a visual impairment struck them on purpose and the researcher inquired as to their response, classmates tended to justify the behaviour of this child saying, "They couldn't see what they were doing." When assured this was not the case, most seemed troubled by the notion of having to strike this child back. Those who admitted they would reciprocate assured the researcher they wouldn't "hit as hard." Responses during interviews were consistent with those observed on the playground. "Paying back" a classmate who was visually impaired created a dilemma for classmates. Thus, in general, peers of the students who were visually impaired perceived these children not only to have immunity from "being picked on" by virtue of their visual impairment but unlikely to initiate aggressive actions on purpose.

Another issue associated with the failure to reciprocate actions of peers by students with a visual impairment was in relation to making eye contact during conversation. Peers of the student with a visual impairment perceived their classmate's failure to make eye contact as a deliberate act of disrespect:

I: *Some kids have told me that when Jamie [student who is visually impaired] is talking to them he doesn't really look at them.*
R: *Yeah, I know. His eyes are going everywhere, they seem in different directions.*
I: *How do kids feel about that?*
R: *I don't know.*
I: *How do you feel about it?*
R: *Well, I think that he should look at you [using indignant voice]. [Grade 5]*

This student did not perceive the child who was visually impaired to be unable to make eye contact nor did he understand that, in fact, this child was aligning his gaze to allow the clearest view of the speaker's face.

Another child expressed a concern that the student with a visual impairment would not listen when they were working together. Because this child did not make eye contact during their interaction, the classmate believed her/his partner was being inattentive. Once again, this classmate had a sense of being treated unfairly because the student who was visually impaired would not reciprocate the same level of attentiveness she herself exhibited during their interaction.

The perceptions of students with a visual impairment regarding reciprocity appeared to differ from those of their peers in three aspects. First, in relation to negative encounters with peers, children who were visually impaired perceived having a visual impairment as responsible for peers not being as harsh in their treatment of them as they would be with other children. As one boy who was visually impaired asserted, "You don't get picked on that much if you're half blind." This reaction from peers was also perceived to occur during positive encounters when peers would do such things as run more slowly for the child who was visually impaired during a game of tag, or throw the ball more easily so the child who was visually impaired could catch it.

The second way in which reciprocation was perceived differently by children who were visually impaired was associated with the "helping relationship" which seemed to exist between them and their peers, particularly in the classroom. Assistance received as a consequence of being visually impaired, such as going to the office to enlarge a handout or helping the child locate something, seemed to be perceived differently than help obtained to complete a task unrelated to the consequences of being visually impaired, such as solving a math problem. In the former situation, the child who was visually impaired appeared to consider the assistance as indistinguishable from the particular activity itself and did not acknowledge, reciprocate, or even thank the peer who had volunteered such assistance. In the latter case, the child who was visually impaired perceived the peer's contribution as "helping" and routinely thanked or acknowledged the assistance in a manner similar to other children in the class.

Finally, children who were visually impaired perceived themselves to have few opportunities to reciprocate assistance from peers. They perceived their visual impairment to be responsible for their slower work rate or their inability to do some activities and were, thus, restricted in the ways they could help their peers as well as the number of opportunities available to help.

Conclusion

Within the context of elementary school pupil culture the opportunities available for interaction between children with a visual impairment and their peers was notably reduced. Without "best friends," they were less frequently involved in more intimate, long-term relationships than were peers who had such friends. Because they frequently were less competent on the playground, they were often left out of activities. The actual process of physically locating playmates on the playground routinely caused difficulties for students with a visual impairment. Such restrictions imposed by the visual impairment were also evident when these students took longer to complete their work, and thus were unavailable to other children who socialized between and during classroom activities.

The quality and/or type of social exchanges characterizing the interaction of students with a visual impairment were, in many respects, different from those of their classmates. Students with a visual impairment frequently appeared more comfortable in their interactions with adults than with peers. Because classmates often perceived it inappropriate to reciprocate some negative actions toward those "who are half blind," students with a visual impairment were considered to be different from other children. Being left to interact with less popular children, younger children, or those deemed undesirable by others, created a dilemma for the students with a visual impairment. They wanted a companion but those available were not necessarily appropriate. As well, routine association with those who were unpopular or, in the case of boys, with those of the opposite gender, seemed to increase the justification for popular children or those of the same gender to exclude them. Since students with a visual impairment frequently received inadequate information relevant to the negotiated rules of pupil culture and limited feedback concerning their inappropriate behaviour, they often displayed behaviours or actions which were incompatible with those considered appropriate by their peers.

When examining the context of pupil culture with respect to the integration of students with a visual impairment, many sources of incompatibility became apparent. Classmates of these students were often perplexed as to how to interact with a student who was visually impaired or how to respond to her/his atypical behaviours or mannerisms. Students with a visual impairment, frequently uninformed of the negotiated rules of school culture, behaved inappropriately. Sometimes teachers unknowingly encouraged behaviours unacceptable to the peers of students with a visual impairment. The social environment itself was often a hostile one for children with disabilities integrated in the regular classroom. Competence, verified in competitive settings or judged on inequitable criteria, routinely placed the student with a visual impairment at a disadvantage. Therefore, it was a complex and often confusing situation for all participants.

Acceptance is obviously a multidimensional phenomenon. For the students with a visual impairment, acceptance was also not a single aspect fixed across time and social context. The same child with a visual impairment who was the centre of social interaction, lively discussion, and boisterous laughter in the classroom was often avoided as a playmate on the playground. Some children with a visual impairment were accepted in varying degrees both in the classroom and on the playground. Thus, their was a complex interplay of attributes associated with the students who were visually impaired, their peers and teachers; the social environment and its many contextual variables; and aspects of communication, both verbal and nonverbal communication, that are characteristic of all social interaction. What was evident after observing at all sites was the need for parents and educators to be actively involved in both monitoring and enhancing the social acceptance and interaction of students with a visual impairment. Suggestions on how this might be accomplished are discussed in Chapter 7.

5

School Culture and Its Implications for the Social Integration of Students with a Visual Impairment

Introduction

The perceptions of teachers, principals, and parents of students with a visual impairment play a significant role in the successful integration of these children and youth. Just as the basic assumptions of pupil culture could be seen to underpin and guide the perceptions and actions of classmates of students with a visual impairment, assumptions associated with the adult culture of schools and those of the educational organization also have a critical influence. In this chapter, adult and educational assumptions associated with the social acceptance and interaction of students with a visual impairment are considered. These educational assumptions are those identified and analyzed in the author's study of the social integration of students with a visual impairment.

How teachers adapt to students with a visual impairment within the specific context of their classrooms and in more open areas of the school will affect their direct interaction with these pupils and, ultimately, the interaction between these students and their classmates. Principals, although having more indirect contact with students than teachers, are instrumental in creating a social environment which promotes the acceptance of integrated students. Given the responsibility of leadership in the school, the principal, through interaction with other participants and parents, can both explicitly and implicitly promote or restrict social integration. Parents, although virtually excluded from the daily interaction of their children within the social environment of the school, provide the context in which early social development occurs. Therefore, the expectations parents have and the opportunities they perceive available for their child may be seen to structure early interaction and thus, behaviour in relation to this aspect of the child's development. Itinerant teachers of the visually impaired, who frequently act in a liaison role between and among the other adult participants as well as between the student with a visual impairment and adults, provide yet another perspective. Given their somewhat "outsider" status and their experience in a number of schools in the same geographic area, itinerant teachers' perspectives represent another source of insight into the social reality elementary school participants construct in relation to the social integration of students with a visual impairment.

The basic assumptions of the adult culture associated with schools cannot, however, be viewed in isolation from many of the constraining aspects of school culture in general. For example, there are policies and procedures developed beyond the school building which have tremendous effects upon those at the "grassroots" level. Priorities of a particular school board or even a provincial Department of Education may be very different from those identified by educators or parents within a given school. Nonetheless, schools must respond and often accommodate priorities, polices, and procedures which originate at levels beyond that of their school building. Therefore, the implications of cultural assumptions associated with school organization and which influence the social acceptance and interaction of students with a visual impairment will also be considered in this chapter.

Assumptions of Adult Culture Relevant to Social Integration

For both educators and parents of children with a visual impairment, integration creates some unique challenges without simple solutions. For example, how does one respond to mannerism such as hand flapping as an expression of excitement by a child who is blind when this has a rather bizarre appearance to other people? Or, how does a teacher include a student with a severe visual impairment in an activity which requires accurate visual interpretation of fine details? Based on research findings of this study, the challenges and questions were frequently different for parents and teachers, given the distinct contexts of home and school. Yet, the complexities and resulting contradictions in some solutions were common to both home and school situations. Both struggled with the concept of "being different" and the negative connotations that holds in our society. Both simultaneously grappled with the need to "make the child fit in" while trying to avoid treating the child differently. As the following adult assumptions associated with the social acceptance and interaction of children with a visual impairment are presented, the complexities created and the contradictions which exist in accommodating atypical situations become evident.

Parents and itinerant teachers for the visually impaired, although intimately involved with the child with a visual impairment, were "outsiders" with respect to the schools. Because the identified adult assumptions emerged primarily from observation and interviews in the schools, the perceptions of these two "outside" groups sometimes differ somewhat from those more directly involved in the daily school life of students. The perceptions of these "outsiders'" sometimes provide an insightful contrast to those of the other adult participants.

Adult Assumption 1: *Teachers ought to focus instruction upon the cognitive development of students who are visually impaired and not upon their social/emotional growth or affective development*

At all five schools, teachers, principals, and parents perceived the academic performance of the child with a visual impairment to be the most important aspect of the child's educational placement. Teachers were concerned primarily with how this student would cope with the academic work, who would provide the necessary programs and materials, how they would manage the extra work, etc. The social/emotional development of the child was not mentioned as a major concern by any of the 18 teachers interviewed.

There are several significant issues which emerged during interviews when the issue of social acceptance was raised. First, teachers did not seem to have reached the stage where they felt comfortable enough with their own acceptance and interaction with the student who was visually impaired to become a facilitator of more appropriate interaction between this child and her/his classmates. Second, teachers did not appear to be particularly aware, either during interviews or observation, of what they could do to assist the student with a visual impairment to make friends.

During observations there were few classroom activities or programs which even broached social development issues. Such issues as "friendship" and "getting along with others" were incorporated in the health program at several sites. However, health was also a "low priority" subject and routinely preempted or was the subject rescheduled when time ran out. As reported by other studies examining the importance given to the social/emotional development of school children (Morse, Ardizzone, MacDonald & Pasick, 1980; Sullivan, 1989) such issues receive sporadic attention at best, and are often not considered to be an essential part of the school curriculum.

Parents of children with a visual impairment also did not consider the social/emotional development of their child to be of prime importance in relation to schooling. They perceived the role of teachers in this regard primarily as one of assuring their child was not "picked on" or mistreated by other children. For parents, as for teachers, academic success was the major concern. The following excerpt from a parent interview typifies the perceptions of parents in relation to their child's social versus academic development:

I: *The next question may be a little difficult to answer with certainty, but I'd like to get your thoughts on it. In thinking about Peter as he goes into junior and senior high school, how do you think he will get along socially?*

R: *He won't have a problem socially. I'm often wondering how much he's going to get bogged down with the extra work. I'm kind of concerned about that. I don't think socially...I don't think he'll have a problem. Um, as I say, Peter has the ability to talk and that'll get you a long way in this world. [Peter is on the fringe of most group activities in the classroom and on the playground he is isolated, spending most of his time alone on the swings.] But, you know, I am concerned about the amount of work.*

[Later in the interview]

I: *What types of things have you done to encourage Peter to make friends?*

R: *When he was a little one, I got into Mothers'n'Tots and I took him. You see, he was always on the go with me because he was my only child. It was easy to go. He used to visit a lot of kids at that time and, then, um, after that, I mean, I never really pushed Peter to play with the kids. When Peter was little he always had oodles of toys and we used to find a lot of the little neighbour kids would come at that point to play, because of the toys, I know it was nothing more than toys. After...once he went to school, I mean, it was sort of up to him to make his own friends, and, as I say, I never heard that he hasn't had friends, um, you know, even like on the swing and that, I know there are kids that will save a swing for him until he gets out there..where he's later getting out or something like this, so...I don't know.*

Parents of students with a visual impairment did not perceive the teacher to have a prominent role in the social development of their child or more specifically to be responsible for their child developing friendships or having playmates.

Although itinerant teachers of the visually impaired perceived the limited social acceptance of these students to be a significant problem, they recognized and were frequently frustrated by the emphasis on academic achievement as the primary goal within the school systems in which they worked. This is evident in the following excerpt from an interview with an itinerant teacher:

I: *What do you see as the teacher's role in the social integration of a student with a visual impairment?*

R: *Well, I think that the role of the classroom teacher, all the teachers, with respect to the social integration of the visually impaired student is actually no different than it is for any other student..whether they are handicapped or not. I think that, if they're, depending on the teacher and the attitude, if they're conscious and compassionately aware of students socially, then they will enhance an environment that will allow participation..and promote participation of the visually impaired student. But that's very, you know, totally dependent on the teach..the individual teacher's conscious awareness. But I don't think that a teacher is going to be, or even, I suppose I shouldn't say should be, any more aware of a visually impaired student's social interaction than other students' social behaviours.*

I: *You mentioned "compassionately aware." You've been teaching for 18, 19 years?*

R: *Umhmm.*

I: *In your experience in the public schools, are teachers compassionately aware of the social interaction of their students?*

R: *I would say overall, no. They're not. Teachers are generally concerned with the academic skills and the responsibility of instilling these academic skills so they can be accountable and be seen to be qualified for their position. But I think the social, generally, the socialization of students, for the majority of teachers, is at the bottom of their priority list, unless it's in the kindergarten program. But, I'm not saying that for all teachers. There are some teachers that are exceptionally aware. And, more aware, so that I'm even at times shocked that they're aware of the importance of social integration.*

I: *Umhmm.*

R: *But generally speaking, I'm talking about the average, I would say no.*

Given the importance others placed on the academic performance of these children, itinerant teachers seemed to have a sense of helplessness or awkwardness in addressing the social isolation of students with a visual impairment.

Two of the three principals also perceived the academic performance of students to be the primary focus of education. They assumed the social/emotional development was being incorporated into the routine functioning of the classroom and when there were problems they "would hear about it." The third principal repeatedly returned to the theme of "the education of the whole child" and emphasized the importance of social development as an integrated component essential to schooling:

I: *What do you see as the principal's role in the social integration of a student with a disability?*

R: *[pause] Ah...one probably in a..leadership role in the sense that, you know, even if there wasn't a handicapped child in this school, at least there's still a primary function to teach caring about others...whether it's in our own community or in the third world, or with handicapped children. And I realize that the one who really makes this go is the classroom teacher. Our staff has a positive attitude about that. I mean, you could make all kinds of excuses why this shouldn't be and that shouldn't be and ah, you know, not too long ago these people, or a lot of handicapped people were simply locked up, ah, and prejudice dies hard. And it can't be a sympathy thing..bleeding heart type of thing. It has to be a genuine concern that this person is going to be a valuable member of society and just as valuable as any other child, probably in many cases will make a greater contribution. And to ignore this child*

> *would be the same as to ignore another child, a regular child. It's just the same as a Grade 1 teacher, like we, ah, she gets 28 children, like in all those four grade 1 classes. Some can barely talk, some can already read, ah, you accept what you've got and you go from where you are. No matter what.*

In all schools observed, the principal's direct role in relation to the social/emotional development of children was perceived to be in relation to disciplinary actions involving children who misbehaved either on the playground or in the classroom. These were the students with whom he/she primarily had direct contact. Even in the school in which the principal acknowledged the importance of teachers attending to the affective development of children, there was no evidence of structured programming to address such development. As in other schools, teachers attempted to address social behaviour which was disruptive to the learning or safety of other students but did not attempt to actively promote social acceptance or positive interaction among students.

As a specific curriculum component, affective education did not exist in the schools in this study. More importantly, it was not visible as an integral aspect of the learning environment. Report cards provided very limited information relevant to the social development of the child despite the fact that it appeared in the official statement of educational goals outlined by the Departments of Education in both provinces. Statements such as "completes work independently" or "cooperates with others" were often the only visible reference to affective education. For the students with a visual impairment, social acceptance by peers was never mentioned in their files, report cards, or on their individualized education plans.

***Adult Assumption 2:** As much as possible, children with a visual impairment ought to be treated the same as other children in the classroom.*

During interviews with teachers, principals, and parents, the importance of treating students with a visual impairment the same as other students was emphasized. To react differently to the child who was visually impaired or to confer other than those privileges perceived to be necessitated by the disability was seen to "set the child apart from the others." When parents met with teachers to discuss the integration of their child, the importance of treating her/him the same as the other children was reported by them to always be discussed. The following excerpts from interviews with parents illustrate how strongly parents felt about this point:

> [Excerpt 1]
> I don't think Mrs. Jones [primary teacher] was the type to ever say, you know, "You guys watch Lisa on the equipment and be careful." Because I think we were quite clear to her at the beginning. At the beginning of the school year I said, "All summer long I will be bringing Lisa down here on

a regular basis to this playground to play." I said, "So by the time this summer comes she will be able to play just the same as the rest of the kids." But the teachers felt it would be different, that there was, you know, when school was open there would be thirty or forty kids on the same piece of equipment. And I just said, "I don't want her treated any different! I don't think she'll get hurt any more often than other kids do." You know, she sometimes, she does on the round-about but it's very rarely on the other equipment that she does get hurt. You know, she may trip over something running along or fall coming out the door but it's, you know.

[Excerpt 2]
What do the teachers do to help him socially? Um..I don't know the grade three teacher as well yet because the year has just started and I haven't met her that much, but...I'm sure that even, like, the grade one and grade two teachers, they treated him as if he was sighted, normal, here comes that word again, "normal." Um, I don't think they treated him any different, at least I don't think they do. They're not supposed to be! [laughs]

Teachers perceived a negative consequence associated with treating the child with a visual impairment differently than classmates. In interviews they were adamant about the need to treat the student with a visual impairment the same as the other children in the class and to allow only those special privileges which were necessary for the student to complete the assignments. This seemingly straightforward approach to dealing with a student with a visual impairment was not, however, as simple as it appeared. Contradictions between how teachers believed they treated the student who was visually impaired and their actual behaviour toward the student were frequently observed. Some teachers were able to perceive the contradictions during the process of the interview, as is illustrated in the following excerpt:

I: *What are your feelings about disciplining a blind child compared to a sighted student?*

R: *I'm about to say it should be the same.*

I: *Umhmm.*

R: *But I can't say that I do, do it the same..as every other child. I feel sometimes I'm more lenient on him. Ah, maybe sometimes he's talking in his group.*

I: *Umhmm.*

R: *And the rest of the class can, see my facial expression to be quiet, maybe. And he can't, so he keeps on talking. And ah, I might say in a quiet manner to him, "Tony, please we're all listening now." But if someone else could see me, if I felt they were still talking I'd speak firmly. I think I do take a little bit more, just go a little bit extra lenient, say, sometimes to his actions or to his behaviour. Sometimes he does get a little bit carried away, too.*

I: *Umhmm.*

R: *Laughing and really getting quite excited about something and, I find there too, maybe..I'm trying not to, I'm trying to show or treat him the same, but his behaviour's not appropriate, but... [classroom teacher]*

The above excerpt exemplifies the dilemma often arising in an integrated classroom where rules have been developed for children who are fully sighted. By accommodating a child's disability in a fair manner, one may be obliged to "treat this student differently."

Principals struggled with similar contradictions to those experienced by teachers when discussing the need to treat students with a visual impairment "no differently than their peers." They too, were somewhat oblivious to their "different treatment" of the visually impaired child as they routinely spoke to her/him as the class filed by, or made a special effort, from time to time, to stop and chat briefly with the student with a visual impairment—actions which were not routinely taken with most other children in the class.

Adult Assumption 3: ***Students with a visual impairment ought to be responsible for making their own friends on the playground.***

Although educators ostensibly supported the belief that teachers had a role to play in the social acceptance of students with a visual impairment in the classroom, they were candid about their lack of responsibility for a child's social interaction on the playground. In general, teachers remained aloof from the interaction of children on the playground except when they were required to address the overt misbehaviour of a particular student. They perceived children to be responsible for creating their own friendships and finding playmates on the playground. The following two excerpts illustrate this perception:

[Excerpt 1]

I: *What types of things have you done to encourage Tony to make friends?*

R: *Encourage him to make friends. [pause] To encourage him to have friends. Like here in their French class? Outside?*

I: *Wherever.*

R: *I don't know [laughs] like, it doesn't sound good does it?*

I: *No, no that's fine. It may not be a thing that teachers would do.*

R: *I don't know, he's just like everyone else. I don't know how you encourage any of them to have friends. [laugh] No, they share, they all clap for one another. You know, listen, I don't know what I did. They're friends, that's on their own, really I think it is on their own. I think, I don't think I do anything to have friends, like I mean I think it's right that they have to listen when someone else is talking or to share, you know, pass things out, but I don't know about, like their friends. They kinda, I think they do that on their own. [French teacher]*

[Excerpt 2]

I: *What is your perception of the social acceptance of Peter by his classmates?*

R: *Ah, he's accepted by them, they don't tease him or pick on him. He, they talk to him and offer to help him whenever he needs them to. He's not really part of the gang. A lot of the kids now have cliques and Peter really isn't part of a clique but he wouldn't be rejected by them if he tried to join them. But they probably don't really ask him to join and Peter stays by himself most of the time and it's really up to him to try and join in activities on the playground. In class he is the first to offer to try something or do something for you but on the playground he's pretty much on his own. [classroom teacher]*

Despite their realization that the student who was visually impaired was "alone on the swings" or "playing with girls from lower grades," teachers did not perceive either a need or a responsibility to become involved in that aspect of the child's social life.

Parents also perceived these children to be responsible for their own social interactions and acceptance on the playground:

I: *How about the role of the itinerant teacher in seeing that the child is socially accepted?*

R: *[silence] Hmmm...the itinerant teacher. She probably works probably more closely with the visually impaired child than even the class teacher in some aspects. Um..I know at least Joan has with Peter, um, you know, although she's only there twice a week, she's still...when she is with Peter it's more on a one-to-one basis type of thing. I don't know, she probably could talk to the visually impaired child if they're not getting along with the other ones and maybe encourage them to take part in more activities and that. You can't really persuade the other way, you can't really persuade the other kids to come back. The visually impaired one has to be able to go out and make his own way, too. She may be able to help that way, I don't know.*

I: *How about the role of the visually impaired child?*

R: *They have to be able to get out in the world themselves and stand up themselves because, you know, it's not always going to be somebody going to look out for you.*

I: *What about the classmate's role?*

R: *Kids are kids. I mean it's nice if they would come and make sure that, you know, that child is involved, but to a certain extent that child has to get himself involved, you know. They might ask the first couple of times, and then if the child says, "No I don't want to," soon they're going to leave him sitting there. But they may ask the first couple of times. It'd be great if they would all the time..keep coming..but kids are kids [laugh]. [parent]*

While teachers were aware of the "different interaction" of the student with a visual impairment when on the playground, parents were not. In general, they assumed their children were well accepted and actively involved with friends during recess and noon hour. Furthermore, as mentioned in the excerpt above, all adult participants perceived themselves to have little control over or influence upon how children interacted when they were unsupervised by adults.

Principals also perceived students with a visual impairment to have the major responsibility for their social interactions. As illustrated in the following excerpt, the principal perceived his direct involvement to be necessitated only when peer conflict was evident:

I: *What do you see as the teacher's role in the social integration of a student with a visual impairment?*

R: *[Pause] To be overly observant, alright? Um, now we have to be careful because...with all adults, interfering with a child's development and their interactions, we have to be careful not to force. What I mean, I guess, by "over observant" is to watch for those things that may be detrimental and to step in at the appropriate time.*

I: *Umhmm.*

R: *If we step in too fast, then we then become part of the problem. Okay? A sight impaired child, or a physically handicapped child, we do not take possession of whatever problem they have. We can't take ownership of it. We can assist them through it, but we can't own it. And once we interfere, we tend to take over ownership not only of the problem it's created, but we then have the responsibility of coming up with a solution. Quite frankly, we haven't got any. Okay? Um, I think we would step in drastically if the impairment, of any nature, was causing conflict in a peer group. That would mainly be the response of the other children. But, again, I haven't seen that in this student (the student with a visual impairment). [principal]*

During the interview, this principal routinely provided reasons why adults should not become actively involved in the problems of limited peer acceptance experienced by students with a disability. As well, the suggestion in this excerpt, of not having solutions to social interaction problems, may contribute to the seeming reluctance of adults to become involved in the social integration of children who are not "fitting in."

In all schools in this study, there was at least one child in each class who was known by teachers to be rejected by peers. This rejection was routinely visible to staff as classmates of rejected children made derogatory comments about the child, tormented and even physically mistreated the child on the playground. Yet, these rejected children were not provided any apparent assistance in dealing with the daily negative interaction they experienced with peers. Adults seemed to perceive the social acceptance of these children in much the same way as they did that of the child who was visually impaired—they were "on their own on the playground."

As with affective education in general, children's friendships appeared to be of little concern to educators. When children were assigned to classes, placements were based upon creating a mixed group of children by ability or separating students perceived to be "a bad influence" upon one another. Thus, class assignments appeared to address the teacher's need for control rather than to enhance the positive relationships or existing friendships of children. Following is the typical response received from principals as they discussed the procedure for making up classes:

> I: *How do you make class placement decisions?*
>
> R: *We make those decisions, ah, every spring. At that point in the year we have a lot of information in the PID file ["Pupils in Difficulty," a file on students who have had reoccurring discipline problems]. We're in a position to evaluate then the additional things that need to be done to assist the kid in learning. We tend to break up unacceptable relationships, deliberately. We do that every year. That's..that's the primary thing that we do.*
>
> I: *Can you give me an example of what you would consider an unacceptable relationship?*
>
> R: *Oh, yeah. We've got a class of..well, let's take the two classes of twenty-four, with about thirty percent learning difficulties. And learning difficulty tends to be exhibited in unacceptable behaviour. Okay? We try..when you get that high a proportion of kids with learning problems..and you're getting kids feeding off of one another.. that's what we intend to break up by placing kids in different classrooms. Okay? Simply to create a better learning environment. So that would be the kind of thing we would do. But we examine every aspect. We do not simply pass a class from teacher to teacher. I've been in schools where that's been done. You know. Just pass them from teacher to teacher. We don't. We spend a lot of time examining the structure of the class, how well it learns, how well it doesn't learn..and try to match those kids up with the proper kind of environment. And I guess that's the only criteria we stick to, is trying to break up unacceptable relationships, with kids feeding off of one another. [principal]*

Therefore, academic and behavioral criteria were the basis for class assignments—not the maintenance or promotion of student friendships or class groupings which would enhance the acceptance of children considered to be at risk socially. When students who were visually impaired were known by teachers to have particular friends, these relationships were not supported by placing both students in the same class. In this study, four of the five students with a visual impairment reported their "best friend" had been placed in a different class this year or last year. For the most part, students' friendships were perceived by adults to be "outside the business of education."

Adult Assumption 4: *Children with a visual impairment ought to have different criteria for peer acceptance than their classmates.*

All 18 teachers interviewed reported that the child with a visual impairment in their class was accepted by her/his peers. Furthermore, several even expressed amazement with the degree of acceptance the student received:

I: *What is your perception of Peter's social acceptance by his classmates?*

R: *I would say it's above average. I think that they...it seems like they socially accept him, you know, more than what if I [emphasizes I] was a kid that I would be likely to socially accept him! But, you see, these kids have had...he's been in their class ever since grade primary, so it's just like, you know, they know that he's handicapped, but they seem to, ah...they seem to accept it and take him for the way he is. Like, you know, if...especially like if...especially if they're playing a game or something and he makes a mistake or doesn't do something right, right? Well, they don't get on his case about it, sort of thing, and give him a hard time, they just sort of accept it. And as you notice, like, they don't, sort of, because his skill might not be as high as someone else's, they don't pick on him. [physical education teacher]*

In the above excerpt, the teacher has based his perception of acceptance of the child with a visual impairment on his observations that the other children "don't get on his case" or "don't pick on him." This was common to every teacher interviewed. The criterion they appeared to use to determine whether the child with a visual impairment was accepted by peers was the presence or absence of overt, negative interaction with other children. The following excerpts are typical of the responses received at every school to the question, "What is your perception of [visually impaired child's name] social acceptance by peers?

[Excerpt 1]

R: *I think pretty good. When I break them up into groups, you never hear them say, you know, "Oh dear." They just treat him like another student sort of thing and I think he gets along really well socially with them. [classroom teacher]*

[Excerpt 2]

R: *Seems to be very good. I don't think it interferes that she can't see that well. As far as music's concerned anyhow.*

I: *What about by other children in the school?*

R: *Well, as far as I know, and it sort of surprises me, they don't seem to pick on her very much, or ah, you know, she doesn't seem to be sort of cut off because she can't participate maybe as well in some things.*

I: *You say it surprises you.*

R: *Yeah. Well kids are very quick to pick up on another kid's shortcomings, and, ah, often times this will get in the way and they'll pick at each other but it doesn't seem to happen in her case. [music teacher]*

The teachers of three of the students who were visually impaired reported frequently seeing this child alone on the playground or routinely playing with children of the opposite gender. This behaviour was not typical of the child's classmates. Yet, they did not perceive such behaviour as indicative of the child's lack of acceptance by classmates on the playground. Even for the boy who seemed most accepted, his seating arrangement in the class with four girls was not perceived to be socially inappropriate. The other boys, and particularly those the teacher identified as his friends, sat together at another table. Thus, in the absence of overt negative interaction with peers, students with a visual impairment were perceived by teachers to be well accepted by classmates.

Parents used the same criteria as teachers to evaluate the social acceptance of the child with a visual impairment. Even in the presence of atypical behaviour, that is, behaviour different from that of the siblings of this child, parents considered their child to be socially accepted:

I: *What types of activities does Peter like to do with his friends?*
R: *They like to pretend like they're T.V. characters. They play with toys. They play Lego. As I say, more quiet-type of play, not a lot of running and that. Even like when they're outdoors running, if Thomas [family friend near Peter's age] is outdoors with Terry [Peter's younger brother], Peter will have a tendency to come back in and play with Mary and show her how to colour and things like this rather than be outdoors running with the boys.*
I: *Who's Mary?*
R: *That's Thomas' younger sister.*
I: *How old would she be?*
R: *Oh, she's four...she turned five, she's just turned five. But he'll come back in and teach her how to colour and her numbers and things like that.*
I: *So he likes...*
R: *Yeah, quieter play.*
I: *When do other children seek out Peter?*
R: *[silence] Hm-m...I don't know [laughs]. Ummm, usu-u-ally [slowly] it's only it's...like as far as home-wise, they don't play with Peter unless they're actually coming to this place, you know; they don't make it a point to actually come here to play with him. Um, at school, I'm not sure how they pick their friends or how they don't. I've really never been able to find that out.*
[Later in the interview]
R: *Peter really gets along well with anybody like that. I mean, you know, he has the ability to talk and I guess, if you have an ability to talk,*

people will listen, you know. In 4H, we find we have a variety of ages, so especially your older kids are very eager to talk to them and this sort of thing, but...I never found anybody making fun of Peter, which I, one thing I probably...at one time I thought maybe I would, but nobody has ever, ever done that.

I: *What is your feeling about his acceptance by other children?*

R: *I think he's well accepted, yeah. [parent]*

Thus, similar to teachers, parents perceived the absence of overt negative interactions with other children as evidence of the social acceptance of their child.

All three principals in this study perceived the student who was visually impaired to be very well accepted. For one principal who had been in the school for only a few months, the criterion for acceptance was based upon information received from his teachers. For the other three principals, the accepting atmosphere they believed to exist for all children in their schools, and the fact they had not been consulted or advised in relation to a behaviour problem with the child with a visual impairment, appeared to be the basis of their perception of acceptance by peers:

R: *I don't suppose I've had an awful lot of very direct involvement with the students who are visually impaired. Again, the attitude here in our school that, whatever children come from is normal..that's probably a big part of what we are, here, with every kid, whatever they come from. It's simply a norm. My involvement, unfortunately, tends to be, with most of the children in the school, when things go wrong. But, I don't suppose I've had any particular interaction with either one of them. They've never been sent to the office for misbehaving. I haven't had to deal with anyone picking on them. [principal]*

The itinerant teachers perceived both the absence of negative interaction and the presence of positive interaction as necessary criteria when assessing the acceptance of a child with a visual impairment. Whether they were more objective in their assessment of this child's acceptance or were, perhaps, more cognizant of the child's feelings in relation to acceptance, having worked with them for several years, their perceptions were comparable to those of students who were visually impaired and their classmates. Itinerant teachers perceived various degrees of acceptance to exist in specific situations involving these students:

A year ago I could have definitely said that he wasn't accepted. Now I'm not so sure. He himself has made an effort to be interested in what others are interested in. I think he's accepted when there's something to do, when there's a task given. And I think the class sees him as somebody who has ideas, has something to offer, therefore, they accept. Outside, I'm not sure whether people actually would include Peter if he didn't include himself. I don't think they'd go looking for his company if he didn't sort of walk up and say I'm here. I don't think they say, "No, you can't," when he arrives and says he wants to do something. I've never seen anybody say, "No, you can't," or "You're not allowed to," but I haven't seen anyone actually go and ask him to join them.

I: *They don't seek him out.*

R: *Well, when he's sitting on the swings, for example, he can sit there a whole recess time and have hardly anybody, except somebody in passing, say, "Hi, Peter," on the way by. And that would be about the extent of it. I've never seen anybody, even if they're looking for an extra in a group, ask Peter to join. I've been in phys ed classes where they've gone through the old two-captain bit and they choose teams, and Peter is always one of the last to be chosen. Um..but I have seen him when it's been a directed activity..when people have said, "Peter, you come in our group." So this leads me to believe they think he has something to offer when it comes to academics, but that socially, on the playground, when it's not a directed activity, he tends to be ignored or left out. [itinerant teacher]*

Itinerant teachers expressed a sense of frustration associated with their belief that social integration would require a "change in the system" as opposed to programs they could do in isolation with the student who was visually impaired.

***Adult Assumption 5:* Children with a visual impairment who are different in appearance should be expected to encounter difficulty with social acceptance.**

Teachers perceived the different appearance of four of the children with a visual impairment to detract from their social acceptance by classmates. In the following excerpts, teachers were candid about their perceptions of the appearance of these children:

I: *What do you think detracts from her acceptance?*

R: *I, I would say...her appearance, I really would. Only because, you know to me as, as an adult and a teacher, I don't mind looking her straight in the eye and I can see, for some kids, it's, it's scary. You know, if you can imagine, they look there and, you know, Lisa's eyes are moving constantly and that would scare, I know it would scare my children. It would probably scare some of the kids in here. But people that have been with her for a couple of years, I know they've grown to accept that. And they just know that her eyes are moving. That's just the way they move. But if you brought in some, a new child, and put them in with Lisa, you know, they would be constantly staring at her. [physical education teacher]*

The "normal" appearance of one of the students with a visual impairment was also perceived to contribute to his more obvious acceptance by peers. His normal appearance was perceived as a distinct difference between him and another child with a visual impairment in the same school:

I: *The next question may be difficult to answer with certainty, but I'd like to get your thoughts on it. In thinking about Charles as he gets to junior and senior high school, how do you think he will get along socially?*
R: *....[Blows out air.] Well..I think there'll always be a problem. Like the other little boy in the school that has visual problems [Jamie]. He looks normal. He bounces around, I mean, I don't know what, how his sight is in comparison to Charles', but, the other little fellow, ah, he's just like all the others. I mean, I don't know how he fits in, I've just sort of seen him out and around on the playground. He seems to fit in a little better than, than my Charles does. But he, I mean, so many people don't even know he has a problem. And Charles, where he is obviously, has the problem, you know, his head is always turned so he can look at, at, out of which ever eye he can see out of, ah...you know, like the scarring on his forehead, ah, the turning of the head, his feet are very toed out, I mean I don't know what that is, that could be anybody's problem, if that's anything.*
I: *Many children with a visual impairment have that appearance.*
R: *It does have to do? Okay. So he is different. And..people that are different are always not accepted as much, as the ones who are, in quotations, normal. And, I mean, you know what kids are like, in the crowds you get in, in junior and senior high school..in the cliques you get in, and if you're not perfect, you know, you're not accepted. Which is not fair, but it's how things work.*
I: *So you see Charles as having problems.*
R: *I think you'll see Charles having problems. And, you know, he'll probably have his own group of friends and they'll be on the perimeters of everything and ah..probably be looked at with, ah, I imagine people will call them weirdos, but..you know, just on the outskirts of everything. [classroom teacher]*

Parents also perceived their child's appearance to detract from acceptance by others.

I: *What things do you feel might detract from his acceptance?*
R: *I think, ah, I think kids stare. They see, ah, some kids are curious. I've always, told Charles to be, you know, to say exactly what, what he, you know, what's the problem and I don't know, I've never heard other kids say, "Well, what's wrong with your eye?" They've asked, people have asked me, but not ah, like I've never heard Charles answer a question like that. [parent]*

This mother's discomfort in discussing her son's appearance was apparent. She seemed almost to have difficulty saying the words "visually impaired." Later on in the interview, she alluded to her son's different appearance and the reactions people had to this. Her anger was evident. Parents often seemed to be tormented by the different appearance of their child. For example, Lisa's bangs were left long to conceal her nystagmus (involuntary, rapid eye movement), although this hairstyle further reduced her visual efficiency. Parents seemed to perceive their child's different appearance as an inescapable symbol of their child's impairment.

***Adult Assumption 6:** Teachers ought not to interfere with the mannerisms of a child with a visual impairment.*

Teachers seemed perplexed when confronted with some of the rather atypical behaviours of four of the children who were visually impaired. Mannerisms such as arm flapping, not facing the speaker during conversation, keeping one's head on the desk, speaking in a voice which was noticeably too loud for the situation, and various hand-manipulating actions were common. Most of the teachers interviewed confirmed their awareness of these behaviours. Furthermore, they reported their responses to such actions to be primarily negative, perceiving such mannerisms to detract, at least initially, from their degree of comfort when interacting with the child. The potentially negative effect on social acceptance by peers was also frequently mentioned. Following are two excerpts illustrating teachers' reactions to such mannerisms:

[Excerpt 1]
I: *When Tony speaks with others, he doesn't usually face them.*
R: No.
I: *How do people respond to this? And what's your feeling about it?*
R: *Well, even myself, I had to get use to it. Because you're use to making eye contact with the person you are speaking to. And ah, it takes a little while to get use to speaking to someone in a conversation and not having that eye contact. A..and with his head, lots of times moving at the same time. Ah..ah, sometimes you're wondering if he's even listening to you. Because that's how you get to know if that person understands.*
I: *Sure.*
R: *Because sometimes you're even noticing the other children staring..particularly the ones who haven't been in class with him before. A lot of them have already had contact with him. So it's just the odd one who has not. And I suppose it's just a matter of..even in the discussion, his head keeps turning quite a bit..and they just sort of stare at him. I'm just thinking of a couple I know who have not had much association with him at all. And they just sort of stare at him, and they're not sure, I suppose, why is he doing that.*

I: *What's your reaction as a teacher, to seeing Tony with his head down on his desk?*

R: *Well..to, at the beginning of the year I thought it was boredom. Okay? I thought he wasn't interested in what was being done or what was being said. This was before I got to speak to the itinerant teacher about it too. But I was thinking that I must ask why Tony keeps putting his head down. Ah..and, at times, also you thought it was an impolite thing for him to do. You'd think you should speak to him and say, "Tony, please put your head up. You're not going to sleep." Which you would do, I guess, to a child who's, if one of my other children had their head down and I was teaching something, I would say, "Jacob, please pay attention here."*

I: *Umhmm.*

R: *And you're almost, I've come very close to saying that, you know, in class, "Please, Tony, you're not paying attention. Look up here, please." And ah, then I, I guess I got over that, and now I'm realizing that he is alert, he is listening. At least that's what I feel. And, that ah, sometimes I don't even notice it now. And I think I'm supposed to be noticing it, more to remind him, you know, not to do it. [classroom teacher]*

[Excerpt 2]

I: *How do you respond to Charles' mannerisms?*

R: *First they distracted me. And really, I don't even think he knew what he was doing when he did it. But it would catch my attention..often. And I just realized that he didn't know what he was doing.*

I: *How do you react now?*

R: *I just don't watch it. I just...keep on with teaching. [music teacher]*

Even when teachers had received information about the child's mannerisms (e.g., Tony's classroom teacher had been asked to assist in extinguishing two specific mannerisms), they seemed reluctant to comply with the behaviour management techniques recommended by the itinerant teacher. Two explanations for ignoring atypical behaviour in these students were common. First, teachers seemed to feel they would call attention to or emphasize the child's impairment by addressing her/his mannerisms. Second, most teachers reported not hearing other students comment upon the mannerisms and perceived this as a lack of interest or as total acceptance. For all but a few teachers, ignoring the child's mannerisms was perceived to be the proper thing to do. This is another example of the contradictions which were encountered by teachers in their struggle to treat the student who was visually impaired "the same as the others."

Principals perceived the mannerisms of students who were visually impaired as an inherent part of the child's disability. From their perspective, such behaviours were either something they would "grow out of" or a character trait which was to be openly accepted, in the same way one might accept another child's unique gait or facial expressions.

Itinerant teachers, as well, did not perceive the child's mannerisms to detract significantly from social acceptance by peers. Although some behaviours, such as not facing the speaker or laying the head on the desk, were reported to annoy them, they were not observed to routinely correct or even be aware of such behaviours.

On the other hand, parents perceived the mannerisms of their children to be a major problem and one they dealt with on a regular basis, as is evident in the following excerpts:

[Excerpt 1]
I: *How do you respond to Tony's mannerisms?*
R: *Depends on what kind of mood I'm in.*
I: *Okay, tell me..in a good mood, and in a bad mood.*
R: *The mannerisms, like what do you mean? Because he's blind? Okay. Some mannerisms, like...flapping, I hate it! The only way to correct it is to keep on his back all the time. My saying is, "Well, I wish you'd hurry up and fly away!" Like, you know, "You're getting on my nerves. If you're not going to fly, then quit." That bothers me. His banging of his hand bothers me. Um, and the only way you can do that is constantly to say, "Tony, you're not to do that!" We used to say, "Your hand is going to fall off," but we don't do that any more because he's wiser and he knows that it's attached and that it can't fall off. Um, they really bother me. [parent]*

[Excerpt 2]
I: *How do you respond to Jamie's mannerisms?*
R: *Well, with these other annoying little ticks, the clucking and the hands and so on I, I'm going to paint his fingers because I think he's going to chew them off to the elbow. Ah...I get...I am annoyed by those things. I really...they're just busy little habits and I just...it's like chewing fingernails. And, you know, I do get annoyed but I-I don't treat him any differently than anybody else. I mean, if Leslie [sister] were doing it I'd say, "Get your hands out of your mouth, please!" The same as I do with him.*
I: *There's a little girl who sits beside him in school. She told me in an interview this morning, "He makes this noise that drives me crazy!"*
R: *[laughs] Well, that must be that clucking. Because he started the clucking again lately, too, I've noticed the clucking's coming back, but the fingers..but they do that. Leslie and John [older sister and brother] had never done anything like that. So...I, I don't know if that...if...and I had spoken to one of the other mothers one night at parent support [support group for parents of children with a visual impairment] about that, especially with the clucking, because it was driving me bananas, and...I don't know what it was her child had done but...ah, it was very similar. It was tapping, I think. Just tapped, constantly. Every...couldn't sit*

down, had to tap. And I don't know why, if that's characteristic of these kids or what. All I can say is it drives me crazy! [parent]

Similar to their discomfort with their child's different appearance, parents were troubled by the atypical behaviours of their child. The "staring public" was an intrusion all parents reported to be unpleasant for them.

Adult Assumption 7: ***Visual impairment ought not to be openly discussed with or in the presence of the child who is visually impaired.***

None of the teachers or principals interviewed during this study had ever discussed the student's visual impairment with her/him. Even dialogue related to the topic during the interviews seemed to create a sense of apprehension. The following segments are typical of the response teachers had concerning this issue:

[Excerpt 1]

I: *How does Peter think of himself in terms of his visual impairment?*

R: *I think just as an ordinary kid. He never goes on about being visually impaired or, beats me, he's just like...if I didn't know he was that way, I wouldn't know because he doesn't show it.*

I: *Has he ever mentioned it in the class?*

R: *No. No, I don't think ever. Yes, I did! One day, I think maybe it was Paula...he mentioned visually impaired to her. It was just like it was a shock to her, you know, to think he couldn't see as well as them...it was like they didn't even know it. And one day, the itinerant teacher was here with a walking cane or whatever you call it? And they wondered why, why was he going with that cane? Just like they didn't know he couldn't see as well as them. And they've been with him all through school. This is the first year we've had two grade 4s. And that's how well he fits in, I thought, because they didn't even seem to realize how little he can see.*

I: *From a teacher's perspective, how comfortable would you feel talking to Peter about his visual impairment?*

R: *Very. He's the type of kid you can talk to. He's so mature for his age, I think. You can really talk about anything with him. Because he always has something to come back with. He's just old for his age. He's the oldest child in their family.*

I: *So you haven't, on a one-to-one basis, spoken to Peter about his visual impairment? [Peter has been in his class for nine months.]*

R: *Not really, I don't think I have.*

I: *I was interested in whether teachers would see that as an appropriate thing to do.*

R: *It probably would be, but I don't try to stress it very much. I just like to treat him like an ordinary kid. I think that's the way he wants to be treated..so let's leave it at that. [classroom teacher]*

[Excerpt 2]

I: *How does Charles think of himself in terms of his visual impairment?*

R: *I'd have no idea. I've never asked him. Yeah, I've, I didn't know whether he, you know, he'd want me to..to talk to him about it or..ah, I guess I've been a little hesitant to, perhaps ask him.*

I: *That's a question I'm really interested in. How comfortable would it be for a teacher to discuss a student's visual impairment with him?*

R: *..Well, I wouldn't want the kid to feel that I was being really nosy. That ah..I mean, some kids are, are reluctant to talk about, you know, any problem. Other kids will tell you all about it. Um..but, yeah, I wouldn't want him to think that I was, being..nosy, just for the sake of being nosy but..and I don't know, I don't know, ah, if, if he's over sensitive about this, or if he would resent me asking..suppose I could have, you know, ask his mother how she thought he would react. [classroom teacher]*

During each of the five, month-long observations, there was only one school at which blindness was openly mentioned in the classroom setting. This was in the school where the student was totally blind and children often made comments about Tony's use of braille or other special equipment. One day during a class discussion about the future, the boy sitting beside Tony commented, "I hope there will be a cure for blindness in the future." Although the other children agreed enthusiastically the teacher was momentarily without words. The following excerpt from the interview with the French teacher illustrates this more open environment in terms of the discussion of visual impairment:

R: *They're all quite supportive, like of Tony. I remember, not this year so much they didn't talk but last year they use to talk. I remember one time Tony had said, "Oh, at home my cousins don't want to play with me. They just think I'm stupid cuz I'm blind." And they're saying, "You're not stupid!" You know, it's really, I was sitting back there just wanting to cry and listening. Trevor [classmate] was saying, "No, you're not stupid just cuz you can't see." He said, "You know a lot of things." You know, and Tony said, "Do you think so?" Sad, oh, it was like I had to turn around to the other side of the room. [She has tears coming to her eyes telling this story.] I really, you know, no one never says anything nasty to him. And he's very smart.*

I: *What is your perception of the social acceptance of Tony by his classmates?*

R: *I think he's just the same as they are. Well, I know they know that he can't see..you know, I'll say, "Close your eyes." And they'll say, "Tony doesn't have to close his eyes." You know? But they don't, you know, they don't push him away. They all seem to, well I shouldn't say they all, you know, it's just the same, everyone has a friend and he can be one just as well as they can. [French teacher]*

Perhaps because it was impossible to ignore the accommodations required for a child who was totally blind as compared to those of a child with low vision, people were less inhibited when issues related to visual impairment were raised.

At one of the four sites, the child with a visual impairmant from time to time announced he was "three-quarters blind." One day during a gym class near Halloween Day, the gym teacher introduced a game involving a dramatic dimming of the lights in the gym. Jamie, usually a competent and very active participant, immediately went to the edge of the gym and sat down. When the gym teacher inquired about this, Jamie said, "It's too dangerous with everyone running. I can't see them in the dim light. I'm three-quarters blind, you know." The physical education teacher appeared both shocked at the boy's frankness and annoyed. In a later interview the physical education teacher expressed his feeling that this was an inappropriate response from the student:

I: *What does Jamie do when he needs help in the gym?*
R: *Ah, he was completely independent in the past and now ah, he still is in his own way. Ah, except when I try to help him now he will say, ah, cute little things, "Well, you know I'm three-quarters blind." [uses sarcastic voice]. Things like this. But as I say, that's just ah, I think that's just a passing phase because he has too much going for him.*
[Later in the interview]
I: *How difficult or easy would it be for a gym teacher to discuss a student's visual impairment and abilities and disabilities with her/him?*
R: *I'd find it ah, difficult ah..to do. But I'd try not to show it. I just try to.."Hey, you're visually impaired. Big deal. Do the best you can." Which sounds callous but it isn't, it's the way I do it. [physical education teacher]*

Although some teachers stated they could discuss a child's visual impairment with her/him and others felt they could not, in this study none of the teachers had, in fact, had such a discussion. Itinerant teachers were the only educators who reported having discussed such issues with this student.

Parents also perceived the discussion of their child's visual impairment to be a difficult topic. They often struggled with this issue and were visibly uncomfortable when it was raised during the interview:

[Excerpt 1]
I: *What does Charles know about his visual impairment?*
R: *He just knows everything. We've told him everything.*
I: *How often does his visual impairment come up in routine conversation in your home?*
R: *..Um, not often, we, we, last year he developed floaters in his eye and it was quite, ah, it was, like it was constantly on his mind. It, it ah, it never, we just always, just if he has homework to do, sometimes I have*

to tell him that he's not going to be able to do it as fast. No, we just don't, if he has questions we answer them but..[silence]

I: *So would his visual impairment or some aspect of it come up on a daily basis, a weekly basis, monthly?*

R: *Ah, no. Not daily, just whenever, he sits too close to the T.V. and I have to tell him to sit back. Like, that's not in reference to his sight, that's just telling him to sit back. No, I wouldn't say, probably not weekly, he ah, he gets headaches sometimes but, ah..lately, well, when he developed the floaters it was, constantly but ah, no, he hasn't spoken about it much lately.*

I: *How does Charles think of himself in terms of his visual impairment?*

R: *..Ah...ah, this year he's realized, I think more that he, he is, you know, with his sight and that, he does know that he is, he is different. But, you know..ah, he, this summer he said he, when he..ah, sometimes when he can't travel like, you know?*

I: *Umhmm.*

R: *He's, this year was the first time he used it. "You won't let me do that because," you know, "because of my, because," I don't know his exact words he used, because you think I'm blind or something. And ah..I told him that he was never [stresses this word] to use that with me. You know, that wasn't to be used. But this is the first year that he's ever used anything like that, he's never ah..never done it again. [parent]*

[Excerpt 2]

I: *What does he know about his visual impairment?*

R: *He knows what happened and...I've talked to him different times. As I say, it upsets him if he, you know. Once you talk to him about it, he's okay. He doesn't know what can cause visual impairment, like with other people. Like cataracts and that sort of thing. He doesn't know that part of it. He knows what happened to him..as best as I do.*

I: *How often does visual impairment come up in routine conversation?*

R: *We don't, never have, hid the topic. If somebody asks about visual impairment and needs here, we've always talked about it. We don't bring it up, you know, if it's just us talking. No, it's never said. But, I mean, if somebody asks or something, um.*

I: *Just in your routine as the days and weeks go by, would it come up?*

R: *No, wouldn't even...maybe, at the most once in every two weeks or so. It's not very often, actually. [parent]*

While adults perceived other children to "never mention" the child's impairment or to seem disinterested, the peers of these children perceived the child's visual impairment to be "none of our business" and were concerned discussion of this topic might "hurt her/his feelings" or "make her/him feel bad." The students who were visually impaired also considered the topic restricted to private conversations with their parents or their itinerant teachers. Unfortunately, this perception that visual impairment was not a topic for spontaneous, candid discussion appeared to contribute to a sense of shame or offensiveness intrinsic to being visually impaired.

It was difficult for adults, particulary teachers, to model a positive acceptance of difference for their student with a visual impairment when they, themselves, were not at ease in discussing or did not understand the student's visual impairment or disability. Most adult participants assumed discussion of the child's visual impairment in public to be an infringement on her/his privacy or to have a detrimental effect upon the wellbeing of the student. The dilemma students with low vision encountered in the nebulous state of being neither fully sighted nor totally blind remained unrecognized by adults and, therefore, unknown to classmates. Given their inadequate understanding, adults often unknowingly contributed to the maintenance of myths and misinformation relevant to the status of the visually impaired in our society. Although adults could empathize with the situations facing students with a visual impairment in a "sighted world," they seemed unable to initiate proactive approaches to minimize or eliminate some of the negative implications they associated with being visually impaired.

Summary

The social integration of students with a visual impairment posed particular dilemmas for teachers, particularly those who had not previously known an individual with a visual impairment. It challenged the ways teachers traditionally interacted with students as they realized their personal and professional goals within the school setting. For example, it was clear in the interviews that teachers considered the enhancement of the social acceptance of students to be a minor aspect of their roles as teachers. They attended to it either in their routine monitoring of discipline or when they observed overt negative interaction among students. Unfortunately, this is essentially incompatible with the social/emotional needs of students with a visual impairment in an integrated setting; they need appropriate, structured experiences to promote positive interaction and the development of a healthy self concept.

In general, children were considered responsible for making their own friends and playgrounds were almost neutral environments for teachers. Furthermore, beyond the realm of the classroom, adults perceived themselves to have little control over students. Since much of the negotiation of friendship occurs on the playground beyond the jurisdiction of teachers, adults perceived interference as inappropriate. Unaware of significant social integration issues intrinsic to pupil culture and faced with situations they frequently felt helpless to address, adults did not take a proactive approach to the acceptance and interaction of students with a visual impairment.

Nonetheless, teachers did not consciously plan or promote the development of negative social environments for integrated children with a visual impairment. Nor did teachers individually produce the contradictions which emerged between the existing school culture and the integration process. As Rogers (1982) stated, these contradictions are:

> *best understood as the unintended consequences of the teacher's attempts to cope with the realities of her situations. It is for social psychologists, in collaboration with teachers and others to attempt to find ways of avoiding these undesirable and unintended consequences. However, this will not be achieved by concentration upon the teacher alone. It has been argued above that the teacher's perceptions of her pupils develop as a way of coping with the situation in which she has to work. It follows then that to understand the perceptions one has also to develop some understanding of the nature of the teacher's situation. (p. 86)*

Therefore, the focus will now be on the contextual aspects of social interaction, that is, those aspects of the school environment or situation which appear to contribute to and detract from the social acceptance and interaction of students with a visual impairment. These basic cultural assumptions are labelled "education assumptions."

Education Assumptions Relevant to Social Integration

Education Assumption 1: ***Teachers of students with a visual impairment ought not to require special training to accommodate these students in their classes.***

During the interviews with teachers and principals, the lack of appropriate training and/or inservicing for teachers who had children with disabilities placed in their classrooms was frequently mentioned as problematic for them. Of the eighteen teachers interviewed during this study, six had taken an introductory course in general special education. Two teachers had attended an inservice specifically addressing the integration of students with disabilities. Only two of the teachers had gone to an inservice specifically designed to address the needs of students with a visual impairment. Obviously, the majority of teachers had minimal, if any, formal training related to either special education or integration.

For most teachers, the limited contact with the itinerant teacher for the visually impaired was their major source of assistance in integrating this child. Each classroom teacher had met with the itinerant teacher and the principal to discuss the student's Individual Service Plan. This is a document written by the itinerant teacher outlining accommodations required by the student, implications of the visual impairment, instructional services to be provided by the itinerant teacher, material and equipment to be provided by the Resource Centre for the Visually Impaired, program adaptations recommended for use by teachers, and any special techniques or approaches to be used when working with the child (e.g., correcting mannerisms). By design, the meeting held to discuss the student's Individual Service Plan is intended to include all teachers who instruct the child and to encompass a team approach to program planning for the student. The majority of the teachers in this study had never attended this meeting, although they may have met with the itinerant teacher on a one-to-one basis. Five of the specialist teachers in the study had never met with the itinerant teacher to discuss the accommodations required in their specific subjects—music, French, and physical education. Thus, understandably, teachers frequently did not feel adequately trained or prepared to meet the challenge of working with a student who was visually impaired.

Few of the teachers interviewed reported having received the level of assistance they felt they required. Specialist teachers in areas such as music, French and physical education frequently expressed annoyance at the limited amount of inservice they received prior to the integration of a child with a disability. [During a discussion of how teachers are prepared for integration]

> R: *In the severe case, we have a boy in grade one this year who is mongoloid and I was terrified getting him. And the classroom teachers always get inserviced to death, but we don't, the specialists, we get nothing, not a thing, which really makes me mad. And our classes are the first ones they put these kids in! [music teacher]*

As mentioned, lack of preparation for integrating students with a visual impairment was frequently mentioned as a major complaint by all teachers. The following excerpts are typical of the responses received to the question, "What guidelines or directions have you received concerning the integration of a child with a visual impairment in your classroom?"

[Excerpt 1]

> R: *That's frightening...I had my afternoon with the itinerant teacher and Peter's mother, but...I did learn a lot there, of course, you would know...black on white [referring to the use of black print on a white background] and things like that. I don't know. Another thing I knew, he had this T.V. thing [closed circuit TV system] and I didn't know how it worked..how complicated was this going to be. But the itinerant teacher was great. She found this desk and she got everything all set up and...like that.*
>
> I: *What would a classroom teacher like to happen before getting a student like Peter?*
>
> R: *I would like to have had the chance to go somewhere and see someone teach. Maybe not...I wouldn't want..maybe not totally blind..well, that, too. I'd like to see someone teach someone at the same level of ability as Peter to see what they're doing and how they teach and how the child reacts to the teacher and his peers. Because I thought, "What are the kids going to say to him? What's he going to do?" And..you know. I just did not know [emphasizes]. I was walking into this blind! But I just learn day by day. [classroom teacher]*

[Excerpt 2]

> R: *What guidelines? [pause] Nothing, I think I came in September, and I don't know, I can't even remember anyone telling me there was a visu-*

ally...I don't know if I asked if something was wrong, if he had a problem, or..nothing.

I: *So there was never a meeting called about it.*

R: *Not that I was involved in. [annoyed voice] [French teacher]*

[Excerpt 3]

R: *And from the itinerant teacher, he has helped me. What to expect, what are some of the habits that he shouldn't do, or how to help him, try to encourage him to do this or whatever. So from the itinerant teacher, I have. And, let me think, guidelines on helping him?*

I: *Guidelines and directions.*

R: *I guess that's..mainly it. The itinerant teacher is helping me now with the abacus, so that I can help Tony with it and understand how to use it.*

I: *What about guidelines for other children with disabilities that you've had in your classroom?*

R: *None*

I: *So since this district has taken on the mandate of integration ["total integration" regardless of the type or severity of the handicap], do they inservice teachers or..[interrupts]*

R: *Ah, well, as I say, the year that this child came in [Last year she was given a student with a severe behavioral disorder.], I was just told that I was going to have him. There was not a choice..oh, inservice you mean?*

I: *Umhmm.*

R: *Oh, no, I can't say there has been much inservice on integration! [classroom teacher]*

These excerpts demonstrate the incongruence between the espoused value that teachers should have special training to successfully integrate students with a visual impairment and the basic assumption that they "ought not to require special training." Yet, although all teachers expressed concern about their need for such training, none had initiated action to receive it. For example, the classroom teacher at one school reported she had purposefully not read the information she was given about Jamie, his visual impairment, and its educational implications because she believed this knowledge would have biased her perceptions and, perhaps, would have resulted in negative consequences for this student.

During observations the effect of teachers having inadequate preparation before enrolling a student with a visual impairment was frequently apparent in relation to both the child's academic and social development. Teachers routinely assumed the student with a visual impairment had access to information he/she could not see, or assumed the use of an adaptive aid provided the same quality of visual presentation to this student as was available to students with full vision. The following excerpt is indicative of the degree of misunderstanding which occurs when teachers were poorly prepared for the integration of a student with a visual impairment:

R: *I've found it kind of hard because I'm only in there once in a while. The only things I really try..I just try to stay around [means stay in proximity of the student who is visually impaired], and I know that he doesn't do as well in French as he does in other subjects, so I just figure that, you know, if I had all these special things I could use and I knew his problem, I could do more, but I don't really know myself what else I could do besides trying to be close to him so he can see what I have and understand what I'm doing.*

[later in the interview]

I: *What were your feelings when you first learned you would have a student with a visual impairment in your class?*

R: *I was wondering how I would do because I knew mostly my subject was visual. So I was sort of hoping that he would be able to work it out on his own. Because I also know, like, I just zoom in and out, and I don't have lots and lots of extra time for those things. So he seems to be doing all right, but I would have to wonder if I had a totally blind...how that would work out. [French teacher]*

A final indicator of the degree to which preparation of teachers for accommodating a student with a visual impairment was neglected was epitomized when substitute teachers were assigned to these classes. Substitute teachers were required in four of the five classrooms during the periods of observation. In three of the four cases, substitute teachers were unaware of the presence of a student with a visual impairment and were incidentally informed, usually by the students, during some part of the school day. At the fourth site, the substitute teacher was aware of the presence of a student with a visual impairment but not his needs or use of specific accommodative equipment and materials. In the following excerpt, the perception of a classmate of the student with a visual impairment exemplifies the consequences for this student of having inadequately prepared teachers:

I: *What are some of the things you would like your teachers to do for Peter?*

R: *A substitute or Mr. Coates?*

I: *Either.*

R: *Substitute..not to treat him differently cuz if...I think it'd feel..pretty embarrassing for him, like if, when they ask him stupid questions or give him too much special attention that he knows, when he knows stuff already. Like, just stupid things..that makes you feel weird and he wouldn't like that. Mr. Coates knows..like at the first of the year he didn't know too much. But now, like, he knows about Peter and what he can do and what he can't do and stuff. And he stops and listens to Peter most of the time, so Peter...so Peter..he can hear what Peter thinks*

> *about it, to make sure that he doesn't get off track and then had to do it all over cuz it takes him quite a while to do his work and he can't be expected to do it more than once! [classmate, Grade 4]*

A final feature associated with the assumption that teachers of students with a visual impairment ought not to require special training to accommodate these children in their classes was a prevalent belief that "a good teacher" could naturally address the needs of these students. Teachers, itinerant teachers, and parents alike, routinely identified the skill of the classroom teacher as being of major importance in the success of the integrated child. The following example exemplifies some of the facets of this belief:

I: *What do you see as the advantages and disadvantages for the student with a visual impairment in the regular classroom?*

R: *[pause] Again, I think, the teacher has a lot to do with it. How much work or how much help she is able to give the child, more so on an individual basis. How far she is prepared to go with, I think, acceptance and extra work and extra help. I, really, again don't have that many problems with it. He's not..you know, they've never had to make major adaptations for Jamie, so I've really not dealt with anything really major. He's had good teachers right up. He's been fortunate.*

I: *I've noticed during my research that sometimes the classroom teachers are specifically chosen for the student who is visually impaired.*

R: *I know, I noticed that, too. Jamie had the most wonderful year in grade three with Mr. Smith. And I thought, "How will he ever survive that year with a male teacher?" Because he hadn't had a male teacher up to that point..and I didn't know Mr. Smith from the man in the moon. And it was the best year that he has ever had. Mr. Smith was one of the most caring and wonderful teachers that I have met. A soft, gentle, gentle person and so soft and gentle with Jamie. And I feared that year would be a bad one, with a male teacher, and it turned out just the opposite. It was absolutely wonderful! And I, I really do feel that for a lot of the integrated kids..it really depends on the teacher. [parent]*

When "good teachers" were expected to be able to automatically meet the needs of students with a visual impairment, the fear of failing this student, expressed by several teachers, seemed to be a realistic pressure and source of anxiety for them. The teachers' limited specific training in the techniques and implications of educating a student with a visual impairment did little to affirm their confidence. Without having received specific training with regard to the potential implications of visual impairment on the social, cognitive, and physical development of these children, teachers struggled and frequently questioned their capability of meeting the challenges associated with meeting the needs of these students.

Education Assumption 2: *The effectiveness of the integration of students who are visually impaired in the regular classroom ought not to be evaluated.*

Since the formal integration of students with a visual impairment, there has been limited research evaluating the effectiveness of this process. Factors which contribute to or detract from the student's learning have not been clearly identified by educators. The degree to which public school teachers are able to accommodate the learning needs of children with a visual impairment have rarely been assessed. Furthermore, the degree of social integration experienced by students with a visual impairment is not routinely examined.

In this study, none of the teachers interviewed had been involved in a formal evaluation of integration for either the student who was visually impaired or other students with disabilities they had taught. Perceived as lack of interest by administration or a situation beyond their control, the absence of evaluation did little to promote integration as an important educational process. The following excerpt, typical of all sites, presents the perception teachers held in relation to this matter:

I: *How effective do you think the integration program is?*
R: *For him [student who is visually impaired] specifically?*
I: *Umhmm. Or the whole integration process in your district.*
R: *Well, again, I think for situations like that with Tony [student who is visually impaired], fine. You know, I think that we got support. We're very fortunate here, I mean, Margaret [resource room teacher] is very supporting...helpful in anything I need. And Chris [itinerant teacher], he'll help me whenever I have a problem. So I mean, I find Tony is well looked after. I don't know if a person who is hearing impaired, or whatever has as many resources. But I find, for Tony, he has, we have enough resources to get him through. Now ah, I don't feel there's enough on the other hand, I don't feel maybe that there's enough, ah..let's see...who's the director or coordinator of student services [doesn't know the name of her district's special education coordinator]? There ah, anyway, maybe it would be better if we had someone coming in to check up on us, like, "Well, Susan, how do you feel? Are there any problems?"*
I: *Umm.*
R: *Yeah. "How do you feel Susan? Do you feel this is working? What is your reaction to having, so and so in the classroom?" You know, or, "Are there, or is there anything that we can help you with that you feel...," you know, I find that, for a lot of it, it's just, "Here he is." That's it! [classroom teacher]*

None of the 18 teachers interviewed had ever had an administrator trained in the education of the visually impaired, local school board special education administrators, or the principal of the school observe their classes to assess the performance of the student with a visual impairment or to provide the teacher with feedback relative to their effectiveness in meeting the special learning needs of the student. Teachers seemed reluctant to seek out such assistance, perhaps because they believed it would detract from their perceived competence. The inadequate evaluation of integration of students with a visual impairment raises concerns about how administrators make decisions critical to the education of students with disabilities, their placements, and their academic and social development.

Education Assumption 3: *Children with a visual impairment ought to be less valued as students than are their classmates who are fully sighted.*

While most teachers did not voice opposition to having a student with a visual impairment in their classroom, neither did they express enthusiasm, a feeling of happiness to have this child, or a sense of executing the child's rights by having her/him enrolled in the regular classroom. There was more a sense that "nobody minded" having a student with a visual impairment in their classroom for one year. This sense is exemplified in the following excerpts taken from interviews at various sites and with a variety of teachers as they responded to the question, "What do you think is the feeling of staff of this school, in general, to having a child with a visual impairment in their class?"

[Excerpt 1]

R: *I don't think it matters much as long as there's someone there to do the extra work and provide the materials and things that Peter needs. Teachers can't be expected to do all this extra stuff, particularly in this day and age where there are so many behaviour problems and social problems. There's no way teachers can do it. So as long as there's someone hired, an aide or someone who's going to do the extra stuff that has to be done for Peter, there's really no problem. I guess I'm not telling you anything that other teachers haven't told you. I think pretty much this is how most teachers feel. [music teacher]*

[Excerpt 2]

R: *Positive. You can ask them but..you know, there'd be a little bit of..this is a little bit different and that, but I don't think there's anybody who'd say, "Oh, I can't do that". They may say, "Oh, I wish somebody else would take him." Ah, there may be a little there, but I think for the most part it would be willing acceptance. Talk to them individually and for the most part they would pretty well confirm that. [principal]*

[Excerpt 3]

R: *At first I thought, "Oh, god, all this extra work. What am I going to do!" [Says in a loud dramatic voice.] I can't keep up with it now. But I, the itinerant teacher has been just super. She came in before the end of the year and said, you know, "You're going to have Jamie," and "What books are you going to use?" And so on and so forth. And I know when*

I have a problem, if one came up, that I'd get help. Yeah, I don't mind having Jamie. [classroom teacher]

[Excerpt 4]
R: *I don't think it bothers anybody. [classroom teacher]*

Another aspect contributing to the perception that students with a visual impairment were devalued was the frequent limited availability of textbooks and instructional materials in a format which was accessible to the student. The following excerpts from interviews and observation notes attest to the frequency and resulting frustrations associated with lack of provision of basic materials:

[Excerpt 1]
[The children have gone to the library for their weekly selection of books.] Mrs. Fraser comes over to help Tony with his selection. He asks, "Are you allowed getting books from down here?" He means the bottom shelf. She replies in the affirmative. He asks Mrs. Fraser why they don't have any braille books in this library and she responds, "I guess they don't have any yet." She takes Tony to another section of the library and they reappear several minutes later with a book Tony has decided on. One of the children asks how Tony will read it because it isn't in braille and Mrs. Fraser replies his mother will read it to him. Earlier in the class Mrs. Fraser had reminded the children to choose at least one book they could read themselves. [observation notes]

[Excerpt 2]
I: *What is the most difficult aspect of having Tony in your class?*
R: *Um..off-hand, I would say, it's all right if he has all the textbooks done in braille. It would be trying to find the time to..help him..if it's, if he doesn't have the textbook, to help him do the same thing as the other children are doing. And with as little commotion as possible. [classroom teacher]*

As evident in the above excerpts, there is a sense of tension here, a contradiction—they "don't mind" yet they "do mind the extra bother." This sense of "nobody minds" having a student with a visual impairment integrated in their class, interrelated with frustrations surrounding extra work and unavailable materials seemed to permeate to the students as well. The following responses were typical of those received from upper elementary children who had spent several years in the same class with a student who was visually impaired:

[Excerpt 1]
I: *Tell me how kids in your class feel about working in school with Peter.*
R: *Well, they don't care because...he's really nice. They don't mind working with him.*
I: *Tell me how they feel about playing outside with him.*

R: *Well, they don't mind. Like, they'd play, if they didn't have anybody else. Like, they'd let him join in a game of tag, or swinging, like, people would give him a swing. Like, if all the swings were filled, they'd give him one. [classmate]*

[Excerpt 2]

I: *Tell me how kids in your class feel about having Jamie in their class?*

R: *Well, doesn't..they don't really mind at all. [classmate]*

By the upper elementary grades, classmates of students with a visual impairment seemed to have developed a sense of indifference to their association with this child. They appeared to have learned to tolerate rather than to accept.

Education Assumption 4: ***Teachers ought not to be involved in the planning or implementation of the integration of children with disabilities in the regular classroom.***

During interviews with teachers it became evident that they were given an opportunity for little, if any, input into the planning and implementation of integrating students with a visual impairment; nor did they demand or request such involvement. The procedure common to all schools began with the principal selecting a particular grade level teacher, if there was more than one class at that particular level. At one site the resource room teacher was also involved in identifying the most appropriate teacher for the student who was visually impaired. Following the selection of a teacher, he/she was advised of this child's placement and a meeting with the itinerant teacher for the visually impaired was usually scheduled. The selection of teachers was frequently made late in the school year, hence, little time was available for preparation or accessing needed training for the next year's teachers. None of the teachers in this study had been given the opportunity to spend time observing the student who was visually impaired prior to the child's placement in her/his classroom; nor had they requested to do this. The following excerpts reveal the limited planning role played by teachers in implementing integration, as well as the level of frustration frequently resulting:

[Excerpt 1]

I: *What guidelines or directions have you received concerning the integration of students with disabilities in the regular classroom?*

R: *[pause and laughs] Haven't had any. I don't know, really.*

I: *Some teachers have told me integration has been imposed on them and others feel they've had direct input into the process. How do you feel?*

R: *Oh, I guess I can say it's been imposed because I've never had the opportunity to say anything, you know, I've never said, "I think it's good. I think it's bad." It just happened.*

I: *You've never been called together to work on how to integrate a student with a visual impairment.*

R: *No! [French teacher]*

[Excerpt 2]

I: *What about the principal's role in the social integration of children with disabilities?*

R: *Interesting that you should ask that question..I would have thought that at the beginning of the year, or somewhere at the beginning when the children [students with a visual impairment] first came to the school, that the principal would have called in all staff members together, all staff members who are going to be involved with that kid..phys. ed., French, so on and so forth, and said, "Okay, you know, this is..," and, you know, just sort of discussed it and everyone shared their ideas about, "No, you don't have to do those things. This is a good idea," and so on and so forth. But ah, I don't think I've had any input that way. The itinerant teacher's the one who's, who's given me the support. [classroom teacher]*

Despite the existence of Department of Education, Teachers Union, and school board guidelines outlining the teacher's role in planning for the integration of students with disabilities, the implementation of most procedures were not apparent at any of the five schools.

Itinerant teachers, as well, frequently expressed dissatisfaction with the lack of input and preparation teachers and they, themselves, had in meeting the needs of students with a visual impairment. The following excerpt is typical of the situations itinerant teachers reported facing in their attempts to coordinate services for the integrated child:

I: *What involvement have you had in the class placement of Charles and Jamie [two students on her caseload], from year to year?*

R: *Um, for Charles..actually very little, very insignificant, other than trying to talk to the principal and to the teacher so, possibly I'd know who Charles might have and what their instructional approach was. Or who either student may have and what their approaches are, the size of the class, etc.*

I: *Umhmm.*

R: *You know, but I found it very difficult in that school, to get an answer, or to get, actually, any concern, any real concern..at the end of one year going into the next year. I couldn't find out who was going to get the student. Because ah, you know, I wanted to know basically, maybe the class size or which teacher would be willing to accept him or, whatever, but, it was hard, it was hard to get a consensus.*

I: *Umhmm.*

R: *For both students. Last year, I don't think we actually knew, until, it was at the bitter end, June 30th.*

I: *Yes.*

R: *You know, almost the last day of school before I had an idea. And that way it makes a problem with ordering text books, what materials are going to be used, and, but ah, you can only do so much. You go to the principal and you ask and you're interested and you try to give your reasons, but, ah, I feel that, there's been, lack of..what's the word I'm looking for? Support, or concern of the principal, on that issue. [itinerant teacher]*

Additionally, the lack of coordination or a team approach to the integration of students with a visual impairment appeared to have a detrimental effect upon their social acceptance and interaction. Itinerant teachers who were only present in the school at specific times had little opportunity to observe the social skills of this child on the playground or during "freetime" in the classroom, and therefore, were not particularly aware of this aspect of the child's school life. When a child had mannerisms which interfered with interaction with others, teachers had not developed uniform, if any, strategies for dealing with these. When a child had mastered a skill in the classroom, other teachers, unaware of the change in performance, continued to provide support the child no longer needed. This lack of a team approach was evident at all schools in this study. Therefore, lack of knowledge, insight and input from educators could be seen to have a negative influence upon the social environment which evolved in relation to the student with a visual impairment.

***Education Assumption 5:** Teachers ought not to adapt their programs to accommodate the student with a visual impairment but should encourage her/him to participate in school activities as much as possible.*

One of the most frequently reported fears of teachers, upon learning they had been assigned a student with a visual impairment, was that they would have to change their program to accommodate this student. However, in this study teachers were not observed to change their programs or, in the majority of cases, significantly adjust their presentation of material or information to accommodate the student with a visual impairment. In some instances this was because the teacher was not aware of the visual abilities of the child. For example, at one school the student with a visual impairment would sit through films without understanding much of the content because he was not given verbal information about what was on the screen. Most often, teachers seemed to perceive their first obligation to be to the children in their classrooms who were fully sighted and seemed to feel they would be denying these children should they alter or adapt the program to make it more accessible to the student with a visual impairment. For example, in the following excerpt the classroom teacher insisted on using the chalkboard to present lessons but did not adapt the approach to allow the child who was blind similar access to information as that provided students who were sighted :

I: *What are the disadvantages for a teacher having a student who is blind in the class?*

R: *Ah..disadvantages..little things, like when I put things on the board.*

I: *Umm.*

R: *Okay, when I put things on the board, say even the lessons. Okay, I'm putting it down for my children to see, to read, and I'm talking about it. Meanwhile, Tony is asking me, "How do you spell that, Mrs. Fraser?" So do you stop to help one, or you say, "Just a minute Tony?" Which one do you put on the side? And, another thing might be..oh, yes, because of the apparatus he has, it does make a noise. Okay, when I'm doing mental math and I want things to move along, it just seems forever just to even get the number one done. You know, and it still..but they're just little things that are like other things, I mean, after a while you learn to work around it..and try not to let it interfere. Like now, today, when I put the lessons down, I think he might have called out, "How do you spell the word "library"?" Well, as soon as he did that one of the kids, Virginia, came over and said, "Do you want me to take my spelling book over and help him?" [Note: The student who was blind did not have the word list which had been provided to his classmates.] [classroom teacher]*

To provide access to the information for the student who was blind the teacher could have spelled aloud as she wrote words on the board or had the itinerant teacher prepare the list in advance—minor adjustments but a definite change to the technique routinely used. However, more importantly, this excerpt suggests two significant considerations confirmed in many other instances during interviews and observations. First, students with a visual impairment were expected to "get what they could" from lessons presented to the class as a whole. Second, Tony is not considered to be "one of my students" but one who has been granted a special privilege by being enrolled in a regular classroom.

As teachers talked about having a student with a visual impairment in their classrooms there was a sense that they felt they should "do as much as possible" to accommodate the child but it was beyond their responsibility to make major adaptations or to individualize instruction for the student. The tensions and contradictions evident in "teachers' talk" are important to note as they reflect the confusion and complexities inherent in the integration of students with a visual impairment. The following excerpts are examples of situations which were routinely observed and/or reported during the study:

[Excerpt 1]
Mr. Coates presents a health lesson. The students are given a worksheet with many small pictures and instructed to find 5 things which would cause fires and 5 which could cause falls. Peter has a lot of trouble finding these because of the small pictures. He struggles through asking what certain things are and if this is supposed to be such and such. He really has to

work hard just to get the information to do this activity which is a simple task for the other students. I notice the children often share their colouring of their pictures with other classmates, showing how they gave this one a punk haircut or certain coloured shirt, etc. Peter has no time for socializing. He works away diligently trying to finish but, as usual, he doesn't finish and has to take it home for homework. [observation notes]

[Excerpt 2]
The children go to music next and sit in assigned seats. At first Jamie is sitting between Ashley and Kevin but the music teacher has changed the seating arrangements. She says, "Jamie, you're supposed to be back there," indicating the back row. Jamie tells her he can't see from back there and she comments this must be an outdated list because that was changed. Jamie asks, "Are you going to be able to change me?" She does and he now sits between Morgan and Michelle and says, "Oh, no! Now I have to sit between two girls." David makes a similar complaint. Jamie puts his head in his hand. The teacher has them imitate some beats which she claps out and then shows them some patterns written on a piece of chart paper taped to the board approximately 15 feet from where Jamie is sitting. He immediately moves up to the board and kneels on one knee to watch her demonstration. Next she says she'll show them some flash-cards. Jamie tells her, "I can't see it." She holds it near him but it is a light orange shade and he tells her he can't see that colour. She tells him she is glad he told her about that and she won't use it again. When she shows the next flashcard she walks away to another area of the room and Jamie has to tell her again, "I can't see it." Michelle also tells the teacher Jamie can't see and as the cards change asks Jamie if he can see each one. After Michelle repeats this question several times, Kevin, who is sitting beside her, tells her to shut up. Jamie seems a little frustrated and sits quietly, not participating for a few minutes. The children are told to turn to page 38 in their music books and as Jamie holds the book to his face the teacher says, "Oh, Jamie, I don't know if you can see that. I'll try to remember to make it larger. I didn't realize it was so small." Jamie doesn't comment but tries to follow along as best he can. He isn't able to read the words as they sing and joins in only when he can anticipate the words from the context. [observation notes]

[Excerpt 3]

I: *When Charles needs help in school or on the playground, what does he do?*

R: *..Ah, I usually see it or have seen it in the past and go up to him and just encourage him and, we've been very honest about his disability. I spent a long time with him..last year, believe it or not, hitting badminton shuttles back and forth.*

I: *Umhmm.*

R: *And he knows he has a problem and I know he has a problem and he just does the best he can and he accepts what little success he has. And it's worked out very well.*

[Later in the interview]

I: *Charles' posture and his toes pointing out, is there anything we can do about that physically?*

R: *I can't and in fact the phy. ed. teacher from the school for the blind came here three or four years ago and was really upset about that. And if I were to work on that then that would make Charles stand out. And the only way you could work on it, in, in the integrated situation would be to make him feel inferior or different. But that's the way he is, you know, Byron had a club foot, that's the way it is. And so, just a matter of accepting Charles for what he is and I assume that his posture, his deviant posture is due to the fact that he's adjusting visually, so big deal. [physical education teacher]*

The inadequacy or absence of teachers' accommodation for the learning needs or styles of the student with a visual impairment had apparent negative effects upon the child's social development. As illustrated in the above excerpts, the student with a visual impairment who had to struggle to see visual material did not have as much opportunity to socialize or enjoy such activities with his classmates. The level of competence was noticeably inferior for the child with a visual impairment when no accommodations were made to enhance her/his performance during lessons and activities. Thus, classmates perceived the student with a visual impairment as incompetent and dependent.

The perception by teachers that adjusting a child's program emphasized the visual impairment was common in all schools. However, teachers also seemed reluctant to provide individualized instruction or to realize that the programs which would accommodate this child or remediate a difficulty would still be appropriate for other students. The fact that these might not be "part of the curriculum" seemed to be a major deterrent for teachers.

As discussed earlier in the text, children who were visually impaired and their classmates interpreted and negotiated meanings related to competence, friendship, and social relationships for themselves and others as they interacted in the context of their school environment. The messages teachers sent when they did not provide equal access to information for students with a visual impairment or when activities weren't adapted to allow for the participation of the student with a visual impairment was obvious to both this student and her/his classmates—it is not important to accommodate the learning needs of a student who is visually impaired, in other words, one who is different.

***Education Assumption 6:** Expectations relevant to the social, cognitive, and physical achievement of students with a visual impairment ought to be lower than those for their classmates.*

Expectations related to a variety of areas (e.g., acceptance by peers, academic performance, independent travel skills) were both intentionally and spontaneously discussed during the interviews and observational periods in this study. For the most part, both children and adults had lower expectations for the performance of children who were visually impaired than for other classmates. Socially, as exemplified in the following excerpts, children with a visual impairment were expected to be somewhat isolated and teased:

[Excerpt 1]

I: *What can we do in our elementary schools to increase the chances of children with a visual impairment fitting in socially?*

R: *Well, first of all we can realize that they're always going to be more on the fringe than in the centre. That's not a bad place to be. I was on the fringe, weren't you? I survived. [principal]*

[Excerpt 2]

I: *What relationship do you feel his behaviour has to his visual impairment or his social interaction has to his visual impairment?*

R: *You mean like as far as being quiet, sort of thing, or to himself?*

I: *Umhmm.*

R: *Just...in a way, to me, when I see him in the playground, he reminds me of a little loner because he just can't participate and can't mingle with the kids the way he would want to. [classroom teacher]*

[Excerpt 3]

R: *I mentioned to my mom one day that I had a boy in my class with vision problems and she was asking me questions like, "Do people tease him?" and that, and I said, "Yeah." And she said that she don't think it's right cuz just cuz he's just a tiny bit different than us, it's just that he can't see. [classmate]*

Expectations were also limited in relation to the physical skills of the student with a visual impairment:

I: *How about on the playground? What does he do there?*

He can't play baseball. He wouldn't be able to see where the ball's coming...or skipping or hopscotch, he wouldn't be able to do that. But climbing on the monkey bars, he might be a little difficult to swing back and you might miss a bar or fall cuz he can't see where the bars are. But he can run through them and climb up them a little bit, but not swing right across. [classmate, Grade 4]

This sense of reduced or inappropriate expectations for students with a visual impairment seemed almost inherent to the schools in this study. It was implicit in everyday activities within the school setting. Following are a variety of excerpts which are typical of the responses and observations associated with expectations for students with a visual impairment:

[Excerpt 1]
R: *Well some people say that you're dumb cuz you're blind or some things like that..you're really dumb, can't do nothing at all. They make up little silly jokes about them like, stuff like that. It's not nice. [classmate, Grade 4]*

[Excerpt 2]
Mrs. Henry, the substitute teacher and the class discuss the story they read yesterday in their readers. Mrs. Henry has the helpers for the week passing out the workbooks and tells the children to open to page 42. As Lisa sits waiting for her workbook, Mrs. Henry asks the class, "Does Lisa have a workbook, too?" [observation notes]

[Excerpt 3]
I: *What do you see Peter doing as an adult?*
R: *Gee, I don't know. Well, there's lots of things he can't do, like medicine.. gee, that's a hard question. Let me think. It's been a long day. I'm having a hard time with this one. He'll have to do something. Peter's too smart to just do nothing. [pause] Gosh, he could probably...teach maybe, oh, there are so many career choices out there now I don't even know about. I guess he's limited to a lot of things, there must be something he'll be able to do. I can't really think of anything right now. That's a hard question. [music teacher]*

As teachers, parents, and classmates of integrated students with a visual impairment experienced the presence of this child, they developed perceptions and negotiated ways of responding to situations which were unfamiliar. Even amidst obvious displays of competent performances by children who were visually impaired, appropriate expectations for them were frequently absent. For students with a visual impairment, these negative messages, both explicit and implicit, were encountered daily as they interacted in the home and school. It is not surprising that the children who were visually impaired came to perceive themselves as less desirable as a friend, less competent, and more dependent than their classmates.

Conclusions

Based upon analysis of data from this research, it was apparent that in many respects students with a visual impairment faced a potentially hostile social environment when integrated in regular classrooms. In the absence of specific training or adequate preparation for the integration of students with a visual impairment, classroom teachers struggled to address adequately the basic academic needs of these students. This circumstance in conjunction with the minimal responsibility educators assumed for the affective development of students, in general, created a social environment which appeared to blatantly ignore the obvious social interaction and acceptance difficulties these students encountered. Furthermore, without a formal, organized plan for implementation, evaluation, and resulting adjustments to the integration process, or even a team approach at the school level, (i.e., a commitment to successful integration) educators were not aware, hence were not challenged, to address the numerous incompatible aspects between existing school culture and the integration process. Thus, the social environment structuring the interaction among participants was one in which tensions, contradictions, and dilemmas were routinely experienced. Unquestionably, the potential for a supportive social environment for the integration of students with a visual impairment was evident. Unfortunately, it was too often neglected amidst the more prominent, immediate, and demanding events characteristic of elementary schools. How the types of cultural assumptions discussed in the previous chapters affected students with a visual impairment will be examined in the final chapter of this section.

6

Cultural Assumptions and Their Implications for the Developing Self-Concept of Students with a Visual Impairment

Introduction

How do students with a visual impairment perceive fully sighted classmates? How do they perceive themselves in relation to their classmates? What are their perceptions associated with aspects of pupil culture relevant to social interaction and acceptance? Answers to such questions were explored through the use of qualitative research in order to better understand how students with a visual impairment construct their social reality. Since knowledge is viewed as personal, subjective, and unique, it is important to understand how students with a visual impairment perceive their acceptance by and interaction with their peers. As well, since an individual's self-concept is believed to evolve, in part, through social interaction, an exploration of the perceptions of these students will foster an understanding of the potential influence an integrated setting may have on their affective development. A critical question is, "Does an integrated setting enhance the development of a positive self-concept for students with a visual impairment?"

Perceptions of Visual Impairment Held by Children With a Visual Impairment

Discussing their visual impairment was a serious undertaking for four of these five children. Even though this topic was not introduced until the second time they had been interviewed and they seemed well at ease with the interviewer, having known her for several weeks, when discussing their visual impairment a sense of uneasiness and melancholy appeared to overcome each child. In the following excerpt, the reaction of a child with a visual impairment to the discussion of his visual impairment was a dramatic change from his usual congenial, conversational style:

I: *The next questions I have, are about your visual impairment.*
R: *Yeah. [quiet voice]*
I: *Tell me about your visual impairment.*
R: *Well, I was born, I was born with it. And when [clears throat] when I was born, I was born with it and the doctors couldn't, couldn't do anything, and I wasn't able to a, walk, and let me see, I was not able to a, [pause] like, now I'm able to get things for myself but back..then I wasn't able to cuz my..thought I might hurt myself that's..but now I'm able to do that stuff.*
I: *What caused your visual impairment?*
R: *I was born with it.*
I: *What does it mean to be visually impaired? What is it like?*
R: *Can't, a [clears throat and eyes are watering as if on the verge of crying], you can, [clears throat], you, like you're, you can't see some things or you can see but you can only see things, like, up close or far back, like, like my Mum. She's either near sighted or far sighted. Like without her glasses she can't see some things. My grandmother's near sighted. Cept she holds some things right up close to her if her glasses are off. Like, right up here [holds hand about 3 inches from his face]. She can't see it. So she has to have her glasses on in order to see things, right up close. [Peter, Grade 4]*

At this point in the interview Peter took every opportunity to emphasize the things he could do, as well as to redirect the conversation away from his visual impairment. However, even the discussion of issues related to visual impairment were obviously very stressful for him. Toward the end of that day's interview, Peter was asked about his reaction to discussing his visual impairment:

I: *When I talk to kids with visual impairments some of them tell me that it's easy to talk to someone about their visual impairment and others say it is difficult. How do you feel?*
R: *[pause] I don't talk to many people, just like my parents. That's all.*
I: *About your visual impairment?*
R: *Yeah.*

I: *Tell me about that.*
R: *Because, that is a thing [voice breaking] I only like to keep open in my family.*
I: *I see. Okay.*
R: *But Mrs. Rogers [itinerant teacher] and all my teachers know about it [emphasizes word "know"] and all my friends, but I don't talk about it with them, only Mrs. Rogers and my family.*

A few days later when we were finishing the last of our five interviews, Peter seemed much more relaxed when questions associated with his visual impairment were raised. His explanation is as follows:

I: *When we were talking about visual impairment the other day, it seemed to upset you quite a bit. Today you seem not to be bothered by this at all. What's the difference?*
R: *Because, cuz today, I know you're still on the subject of visual impairment. I didn't know that..you just surprised me with that one. [means he was taken by surprise by the questions on visual impairment during our second interview]*

These children had also developed some confusion surrounding the perception of being "handicapped." The mother of the six-year-old child who was visually impaired related the following story during the parent interview:

> [mother is commenting on society's attitude toward the disabled] These are the 1990s and we are still so unsure of these people [people with disabilities] and we tend to think of them as different, because they have a problem or a handicap, right? And, the first time we went into a bathroom, a handicapped bathroom, [laughs] and Lisa went in there and she said, [in a whisper] "Am I allowed to be using this bathroom?," and I said, "Yes, dear," and she said, "But it says handicapped." And I said, "Honey, as hard as this may be for you to believe," I said, "You're classed in that category." She says, "I am!" [laughs] And I said, "Yeah." But every time we go to the mall, you know, "Don't park in the handicapped zone." And I said, "Never, I would never do that, Lisa." And she said, "How come you can't park there if I'm considered handicapped? Why can't you park there?" Right? And I said, "Because you can walk!" I said that the parking spots would mean for wheelchairs. But it's hard for kids to understand what handicapped means. Because she said to me, "I thought handicapped meant only someone in a wheelchair." And I said, "No. You would be considered handicapped because you have a vision problem." You know. And I said, "Someone deaf would be considered handicapped." I said, "It's, it's all different." You know. And I think it really surprised her that, I would..and, I figured it's better for you to know now than for someone to say to you later, you know, "She's a handicapped child." Right? For her to say, "What am I? What is this word?" [parent]

The child's perception of this same incident was spontaneously related in relation to another question posed by the researcher during interviews a week and a half later:

I: *Who are the kids in your class that the other kids do not seem to play with very often?*
R: *I don't know. Me, mostly me. [says in sad voice]*
I: *Other kids don't seem to play with you? Tell me about that.*
R: *Hard to talk about.*
I: *It is.*
R: *Don't know. It's because I'm handicapped.*
I: *What does that mean?*
R: *Like it's my eye vision. Mum always kept it as a secret. [talking in a low, quiet voice]*
I: *Did she?*
R: *All this time [in whining voice].*
I: *Your mother kept it a secret.*
R: *'Cept once.*
I: *One time.*
R: *Umhmm. Hardly anyone knows.*
I: *Oh, what do you mean your mother's keeping it as a secret? I don't understand.*
R: *She kept it a secret since I was a baby.*
I: *Who did she keep it a secret from?*
R: *Me!*
I: *Oh, from you. When did you find out?*
R: *She told me one night when I was in town with her.*
I: *Umhmm. Can you tell me about that.*
R: *Okay. Um, see well, I was using the bathroom for wheelchairs, the handicapped bathrooms, and then she told me.*
I: *Oh, I see. So did you know you were handicapped before that?*
R: *[nods no]*
I: *Tell me about your handicap.*
R: *I don't barely know anything about it. [Lisa, Grade 1]*

For older children in the study this confusion surrounding the concept of being handicapped was apparent in their perceptions of the actual restrictions imposed by their disability. For example, in the following excerpt Peter is talking, in general, about friends. His visual impairment has not been introduced in the initial part of the discussion below:

I: *What are some things your friends do or say that help?*
R: *Well, they tell me that was a good pitch, like my, Alice, my housekeeper?*
I: *Ummhm. I had to turn the steering wheel in my Grandpa's truck because he got it stuck and he was towing it with the tractor. And he told*

me, "Very good!" [much pride in voice] When I got on that tractor, I was as nervous, I was very nervous, I hadn't droven! I hadn't did that for a dog's age. I had never driven before! That was my first time. My legs were shaking [Arms start flapping in excitement. Peter did not realize someone with a visual impairment would be allowed to do this].

[Later in the interview after discussion of visual impairment has been introduced]

I: *Is there anything you want to do in school, but they don't let you do because of your visual impairment?*

R: *No.*

I: *They let you do anything you want to do?*

R: *[On verge of tears] They let me do anything I want to. But my mum and dad don't let me go out down those streets by myself.*

I: *Oh, yes.*

R: *Because of my vision. Yup.*

I: *Is there anything else either at home or at school that you're not allowed to do because you're visually impaired?*

R: *[pause] One thing I am allowed to do now that I found out...*

I: *What's that?*

R: *I'm allowed to turn the steering wheel in my father's truck. I thought that I was visually impaired, that ah, Grandpa wouldn't want me to...that he would wait until Dad got home to help him. Well, he came in and asked me and I found that as a shock! [very proud of this].*

I: *How did that make you feel?*

R: *[in a delighted voice] Surprised!*

Peter's amazement at being able to do something he perceived only those with sight could do (i.e., turn the steering wheel) is noteworthy. It makes one wonder how many things these children automatically assume are beyond their capabilities without ever having had the opportunity to experiment with them.

As the research progressed and other children with a visual impairment were interviewed, it became evident that these children felt a great deal of pressure to be like the other children in their classrooms. Interview questions designed to explore the understanding associated with making and keeping friends that students with a visual impairment had developed revealed the "boundaries" to which they felt a need to comply:

I: *Suppose I was a new kid just starting this school and I didn't know anyone. If you and I were talking before my first day of school, what would you tell me I should and should not do if I wanted the kids to like me?*

R: *You should let them..you should share your stuff. You should learn not to talk out during class. And try to stay within the boundaries. You don't know what that means.*

I: *No, tell me about that.*
R: *Well, stay within in the boundaries means, try and do stuff that they're doing. Like play with them. If you don't want to, like if they ask you to play with them and you don't want to, just say "No, I'd rather play with so-and-so."*
I: *And that's staying within the boundaries?*
R: *Yeah.*
I: *Tell me more things that are staying within the boundaries.*
R: *Like your trying to get as much work as you can done in the school day, so you don't have that much for homework. That's what I, I'm trying to stay in the boundaries. So I don't have that much homework cuz I hate homework.*

Peter's comments about staying within the "boundaries" were common to all five students with a visual impairment as they expressed their concerns about doing what was perceived to be "the right stuff for normal people" and their negative feelings about acting different from those who were fully sighted. Even Tony, the student who was totally blind but who felt the most comfortable talking about his blindness, was reported to experience some difficulties comprehending the restrictions of his disability. In the following excerpt his resource teacher relates one such example:

I: *What do you think will happen when Tony starts to realize, maybe, some of the implications of his blindness?*
R: *Last year the itinerant teacher used to take Tony out for dinner every Tuesday as part of his life skills program. And once he invited me to go along and we were in the restaurant, and Tony looked at me and said, "What am I going to do when I'm 20 and I'm on my own? I'll never be able to live alone." And that really struck a chord with me, it really bothered me. And of course, Chris [itinerant teacher] said, "Yes you will, Tony. You'll learn. We're going to teach you how to do this and this and this." But he said, "How am I going to cook my supper? How am I going to do this?" And that really bothered me.*
I: *Umm.*
R: *Because he was thinking 12 years ahead.*

Again in this excerpt, it is evident that the student had developed some inaccurate beliefs relevant to the limitations imposed by his disability. The sense of dependence on others seemed almost second nature to these students.

As interviews with the four children with low vision were analyzed, it became apparent that they had come to interpret their visual impairment as something that was "bad" or something for which they should be ashamed. Corn (1987) and Mangold (1980) have alluded to the meanings children who are visually impaired construct from the subtle, negative messages they receive in relation to their visual impairment. Children receive negative messages about their visual impairment when parents display disappointment when they cannot identify small symbols during vision tests, when well-intentioned adults ask, "What's *wrong* with his vision?", when teachers express their frustrations because the child cannot see the page being used in a particular activity, and when they are the last ones chosen by their peers as a team member or partner for an activity. The use of the word "wrong" in the following letter, written by Jamie, the grade five boy who was visually impaired, is indicative of the subtle manner in which language affects the meanings constructed. He wrote this letter to demonstrate to his mother some new typewriter features which he had recently learned and spontaneously chose to write about his vision:

> *[Note: The spelling errors have not been corrected] When I was egzactly one year of age they found out I was leagily blind after the test's. Then when I was about three or four years old I had to go to Toronto for more tests. I forgot to tell you when I was two I had a cat scan done to make sure there was not any more wrong. But they said there was nothing else wrong. So now my decrease is better than what it had been. But my sight has not changed and now I am in grade five and I love using my typewriter and the computer. I hope my eyes get better.*

All of the children with a visual impairment in this study attributed their exclusion from particular activities by their peers to their visual impairment. Even the child who was routinely uncooperative with peers and teachers reported the visual impairment to be the grounds for the rebuffs received from some peers. The potency of being visually impaired on the self-concept of these children is exemplified in the following excerpts—the first, in which visual impairment is perceived to have a positive impact upon popularity, the second, in which it is perceived to have a negative effect:

[Excerpt 1]
R: *I'm pretty popular.*
I: *What makes you popular?*
R: *Cuz people like me.*
I: *Why do people like you?*
R: *I don't know, because I'm blind maybe.*
I: *Is that why they like you?*
R: *I don't know, yeah, probably. [Tony]*

[Excerpt 2]
I: *What do your friends know about your visual impairment?*
R: *Not much.*
I: *Can you think of anyone who knows anything about it?*
R: *Well, you know that girl I was telling you about? [a girl in grade 6] She just doesn't like it.*
I: *She doesn't like your visual impairment? [nods yes] The one in grade 6. How do you know that?*

R: *Why would she try to beat me up if I..wasn't visually handicapped. I wish I knew where she lived. I could tell her parents.*
I: *Does having a visual impairment make it easier or more difficult to make friends?*
R: *[pause] A bit difficult.*
I: *Can you tell me about this?*
R: *You see, most people hate me. Like Billy, he's in the last grade. And he's on my field day team. He hates me.*
I: *Can you tell me more about why it's more difficult to make friends if you're visually impaired?*
R: *Well, it's easier to make friends when, you're, you have perfectly good eyesight.*
I: *Is it? What makes it easier?*
R: *Cuz if someone asks you something far away when you were legally blind and you didn't tell them and they were new? [means new to the school, i.e. a new acquaintance]*
I: *Umhmm.*
R: *Then if you didn't see it they'd know and if you wanted to keep it a secret...*
I: *Do you want to keep it a secret?*
R: *[nods yes] But it just came out of my mouth.*
I: *Why do you want to keep it a secret?*
R: *Because everybody makes fun. [Lisa]*

Having a visual impairment was perceived by these students as problem - atic for friends as well as for parents and teachers. This perception is illustrated in the following excerpt:

I: *Are there other kids in your school with a visual impairment?*
R: No.
I: *Would you like there to be?*
R: No.
I: *Can you tell me about that?*
R: *Because I like friends who are sighted.*
I: *What about those that are visually impaired?*
R: *I do have one friend but he's not in this school. Well, he, well, I'm glad there aren't other visually impaired kids in this school. It would be hard trying to get along with, ah, four visually impaired people, two or, that's as high a number as you can go, two.*
I: *Can you tell me about that?*
R: *Like, it'd be too..kinda hard playing with three or four people at the same time. Like one person that is visually impaired is all you can play with at one time.*
I: *I'm not sure I understand this.*
R: *Well..it's just more difficult to play with someone who's visually impaired. Teachers can't help more than one. [Peter]*

Limited knowledge concerning their visual impairment was another commonality among the five children who were visually impaired. The oldest child, who was nearly thirteen, provided the following information:

I: *Tell me about your visual impairment.*
R: *Well, I was blind in one eye since I was born.*
I: *Umhmm.*
R: *At least I think I was since I was born, then, I think this eye turned or something.*
I: *Oh, yes.*
R: *I don't know. I think they had to put a laser in this one so it would, the retina would stay.*
I: *Oh, yes. That's your good eye.*
R: *Yeah.*
[later in the interview]
I: *What do the children in your class know about your visual impairment?*
R: *They know I'm blind in one eye.*
I: *And what do they know about the amount of vision you have in your other eye?*
R: *They know it isn't much [laughs].*
I: *What's your visual acuity?*
R: *What's, what's that mean?*
I: *Like, 20/20 is my visual acuity and..*
R: *I'm not sure. I think it's 20 over 40, I'm not, I don't know. I'm not sure. Maybe it's five out of twenty or something, I don't know. [Charles' visual acuity was 20/400]*

None of the children in the study gave the medical name for their eye condition (e.g., optic atrophy), or were they aware of their visual acuity:

R: *Jamie, you told me you have some problems with your eyesight.*
I: *Tell me about that.*
R: *Like, how did it come?*
I: *Yes, just tell me about your, what do you call it?*
R: *Oh, god, I can't remember that name. Lazy eye, it's called lazy eye but there's some different title for it. I don't know what that title is any more.*
I: *Do you say you have a sight problem, you have visual impairment..*
R: *Yep.*
I: *You have a..*
R: *Yep, vision handicapped. I'm legally blind, actually.*
I: *You're legally blind. Okay. Well, tell me about that.*
R: *Like, what is it or how blind I am and things?*
I: *Sure.*
R: *My blindness is 20%. I'm 20% blind, I'm three-quarters blind, what am I saying, three-quarters and 5% blind. I have 20% eyesight left.*

I: *You have 20% of your eyesight left. Okay. What else do you know about your visual impairment?*

R: *I was born that way and I had to go to Toronto for some tests on my eyesight. [Jamie]*

The four children with low vision were anxious to assure the interviewer they were not totally blind but had some "pretty good vision." All were aware that they were "born with it" and that their parents "wished they weren't that way."

Peers' Perceptions of Visual Impairment and of Students With a Visual Impairment

Through their observation of and interaction with a student who was visually impaired, classmates interpreted behaviours and formed impressions of the student and her/his degree of social integration. By exploring these perceptions, adults can better understand those aspects of the social environment of schools which must be addressed when attempting to enhance the social acceptance and interaction of students with a visual impairment.

Discussion of the eye condition of a classmate who was visually impaired did not appear to be particularly difficult for the peers of students with a visual impairment. However, one of the most startling aspects of the interviews with the five to eight classmates at each school was their lack of knowledge about both their classmate's eye condition and basic functional implications of her/his impairment. The following excerpts are representative of the responses to the question, "What do you know about [the student with a visual impairment] eye condition?"

[Excerpt 1]

R: *Well, he's blind and...he's, he goes around with, he's got another teacher.*

I: *Mmhm, Mrs. Rogers [itinerant teacher].*

R: *Yeah. And she takes him for walks and everything. Like, he has his cane, and he uses it. And he goes off by himself in front of Mrs. Rogers and can cross the streets now.*

I: *Why are children "half blind"? [Note: The term "half blind had been used by this child in an earlier segment of the interview. During the research, the interviewer used the terminology provided by the student being interviewed.]*

R: *Um, because they, um, don't eat the right..proper, food, like carrots make your eyes see better. They probably don't eat as much carrots as everybody else does, and eat things that are bad.*

I: *Do you know anyone else who is "half blind", who can't see very well?*

R: *No, not really. [Grade 4 classmate]*

[Excerpt 2]

I: *Why are children "half blind"?*

R: *[pause] Um, cuz ah, there's just stuff. It comes from the air and it goes into your eyes and then it makes your eyes blind. Sometimes it goes right through the air and nose bone to this one then you're blind. But Lisa is only this eye blind.*

I: *Just blind in her right eye.*

R: *Yeah.*

I: *Do you know anyone else who is half blind?*

R: *Nope. [Grade 1 classmate]*

[Excerpt 3]

R: *That it might not get cured or stuff. Some people might get a cure for it though.*

I: *Why are children blind?*

R: *Well..well, sometimes you get really sick and get a real bad disease and stuff. And you get, turn blind and stuff like that.*

I: *Do you know anyone else who's blind?*

R: *No. [Grade 3 classmate]*

[Excerpt 4]

R: *Well, it's pretty good. And, like, most of the time he can't, like, see most of the words, and you have to get it blown up for him so it's bigger. And, like....do you want to repeat your question again?*

I: *Tell me what you know about his visual impairment.*

R: *Well, it's...mostly...like, it's pretty good...like, his vision is okay, like, for playing most of the things...like hockey, it's easy because it's black and the ice is white. And like, he can play hockey. And, um, his visual impairment is...like, it's sort of hard for him to see, I'm pretty sure it is. And like, some of the time it's easy for him to see, but I don't think it's that easy for him. Like, he can read his own writing and everything, but most of the time he can't read the teacher's unless she prints.*

I: *Why do children have visual impairments?*

R: *I'm not sure. Like, probably because, like, they were born with it and they couldn't see very well when they were born...so...and, like, they just had to keep it. That's the same with me and I couldn't get glasses until I was two. So...I couldn't see very well until I was two. I can still see without my glasses on. [Grade 5 classmate]*

[Excerpt 5]

R: *Not much of any of it.*

I: *Why are children blind?*

R: *Well, some people are just born that way. Some people play with firecrackers and stuff. They blow up in their face.*

I: *Do you know anyone else who is blind?*

R: *No. [Grade 6 classmate]*

[Excerpt 6]

R: *..I don't know that much. I just know that he can't see. I don't know if he was born that way or if he was in an accident. I don't know.*

I: *Why do children have visual problems?*

R: *..I don't know.*

I: *Do you know anyone else with a visual problem?*

R: *No. [Grade 6 classmate]*

Overall, classmates of the child with a visual impairment were uninformed of this student's condition. There was a tendency for classmates to relate the child's visual impairment to some aspect of visual functioning they themselves experienced, as is evident in Excerpt 4. None of the 31 classmates interviewed mentioned a specific name, medical or otherwise, for the child's visual condition. Students with a visual impairment were generally described as "doesn't see as good as us" or as "not able to see too good." Most often they described functional implications of the visual impairment which they had observed on a daily basis, such as, "has to use a cane", "can't read small print", or "holds stuff real close."

Two of the 31 children interviewed mentioned having asked their classmate who was visually impaired specific questions about what he/she could see in a given situation. These children appeared to have a more specific understanding of the student's visual abilities and difficulties in a specific situation, but still a less than comprehensive understanding of the child and the impairment. Given the difficulties discussing and describing their visual impairment experienced by most of the students who were visually impaired, this might be expected. As well, the reluctance of teachers to draw attention to the child's visual impairment, as discussed earlier, may also have contributed to the limited relevant knowledge classmates appeared to have.

As is evident in the above excerpts, explanations classmates gave for children being visually impaired were frequently vague and based on conjecture. Several children during the interview commented that the child's visual impairment was "none of our business" or that students "don't talk about it." There was a sense that this was a confidential topic discussed only in small, private groups. The majority of children believed visual impairment to be the result of an accident or something one was "born with." Even though the explanations tended to become more sophisticated as the age of the children increased, the reflected understandings were based more on conjecture than accurate information. Several of the children interviewed in the upper elementary grades suggested God was responsible or the child's mother had taken something during her pregnancy. Following are two such explanations and descriptions of the student's visual condition:

[Excerpt 1]

I: *Tell me what you know about Jamie's visual condition.*

R: *Well, he's quarter eye blind in each eye so..*

I: *He's quarter eye blind in each eye.*

R: *Quarter eye blind in each eye. It's like say, right over here to the pu..the middle of the pupil would be blind, he'd be blind. And the same with this eye.*
I: *Oh, so in the rest of the eye he can see okay?*
R: *Umhmm.*
I: *Why do children have visual problems?*
R: *God, maybe that's the way they were born. Or God gave it to them. So they can be special. [Grade 5 classmate]*

[Excerpt 2]
I: *Tell me what you know about Jamie's vision.*
R: *I don't know hardly nothing about it. Only that he needs to use a sth..sth..stethoscope [means telescope].*
I: *Why do children have visual problems?*
R: *Born like that. God wants them to be that way. [Grade 5 classmate]*

Although peers seemed to feel it was inappropriate to openly discuss the student's eye condition in her/his presence, children did make some self-initiated attempts to acquire more information about the child's visual impairment. All five of the children who were visually impaired reported situations in which peers had attempted to test their visual abilities by holding up fingers for them to count or asking them questions which they could use to compare their own visual abilities to those of the child who was visually impaired. Following is Peter's report of such a test:

I: *Peter, what do you say when your friends say you can't see?*
R: *I say I can, part. I say I'm visually impaired. And they'd usually go, "How many fingers am I holding up?" And I'd look and then I'd tell them. Yup.*
I: *And you can tell?*
R: *[in a happy voice] Yes, but now they're starting to get tricky.*
I: *What are they doing?*
R: *Like, they're saying, like, when I tell them five fingers, they say it's wrong. See, they're, they're trying to request four fingers and one thumb.*
I: *Oh, I see. That is tricky.*

The element of teasing apparent in this situation was common to other sites observed during the study. However, the subtlety and brevity of such occurrences seemed to suggest curiosity rather than malicious intent on the part of peers.

There was another perception, common to all sites, related to the understanding peers had about their classmate's vision. This was a suspicion the child with a visual impairment was "faking" her/his visual impairment to get special privileges or attention. Although researchers (Corn, 1987; Mangold, 1980) have described hardships experienced by those with low vision which are associated with misunderstandings arising from the inconsistent abilities inherent with being neither totally blind or fully sighted, in this study even the child who was totally blind was suspected of "playing tricks" and some children queried his visual abilities. Therefore, without accurate information about the student's visual impairment, classmates sometimes appeared to be sceptical of the authenticity or the severity of the disability.

Children's perceptions of the student who was visually impaired were marked by inconsistencies and contradictions. During interviews they frequently described this student as "just like a normal person" yet they expressed a sense of marked difference between themselves and the child with a visual impairment. Children with a visual impairment were perceived to need more attention, receive more help, have some immunity from "being picked on," and generally believed to wish they could see as "good as the other kids."

Knowing the child was visually impaired seemed to have a potent effect upon how peers perceived all aspects of their classmate's performance and behaviour. The fact that their classmate was known to be blind or to have problems with her/his vision seemed to function as a "label of primary potency." In the interviews, before any discussion of the pupil's visual impairment had occurred, classmates reported children liked or disliked the child with a visual impairment "because he's blind" as opposed to character traits such as friendly, generous, weird, or mean. Activities in which the child with a visual impairment did not participate were interpreted to be "too hard cuz he's blind" while other children might be excused based upon likes and dislikes for certain activities. The student's scarcity of friends was explained by "they don't hang around him cuz he's blind" or "since he can't see he goes his separate way." The most prominent perception of classmates was in relation to the amount of help their visually impaired classmate required to complete even routine activities. To be visually impaired was to require routine help from both teachers and peers. In short, the label "visually impaired" or "blind" seemed to dominate the perceptions classmates had of these students regardless of the activity or behaviour they were describing.

Contradictions and Dilemmas Evolving in the Integrated Setting

As the cultural assumptions inherent to the social environment of elementary schools were identified and the perceptions of students with a visual impairment and their peers were recorded, data from the many sources needed to be examined from a broader and more interrelated perspective. In the remainder of this chapter, an attempt is made to bring together some of the emerging themes in the researcher's exploration of the social environment of the integrated school setting and the acceptance and interaction between students with a visual impairment and their peers. The focus is upon the complex and sometimes unanticipated ways in which people respond to atypical circumstances within their environment. These are discussed in terms of: (1) the contradictions which seem to be created within schools when people were challenged to perform in ways which were different from or incompatible with their current function and, (2) some of the dilemmas which arose in relation to the social acceptance and interaction of a child with a visual impairment as other people (children and adults) in elementary schools constructed meanings and adopted strategies to cope with this student. Following this, consideration is given to the implications these contradictions and dilemmas may have upon the beliefs constructed by children with a visual impairment and the potential for them to develop a positive self-concept within the integrated setting.

The Contradictions

The "essence" of a culture, that is, its basic assumptions, are present when a student with a visual impairment is enrolled in a given school and assigned to a specific classroom. Since children with a visual impairment have traditionally been educated in segregated schools for the blind, their enrollment in public schools can be seen to challenge the basic assumptions of existing school culture, that is, teacher and pupil culture. As integration challenges the basic assumptions of elementary school culture, a "new shared experience begins the formation of a new culture" (Schein, 1985, p. 184). However, as this culture evolves contradictions will be evident.

A contradiction is a statement, belief, or practice which is at variance, incompatible, or inconsistent with the general circumstances within a given situation. In this study there were two significant contradictions evident at all sites which appeared to detract from the social acceptance and interaction of students with a visual impairment. Both were related to the incompatibility existing between the philosophical implications of integration and the cultural assumptions currently intrinsic to elementary schools. The first was related to how participants in the study value difference among children; the second was the contradiction evident between the concept of individualized programming and progress explicit to integration and the basically competitive learning environments present in elementary classrooms.

The first contradiction is inherent to the assumption that to be different is undesirable. Integration assumes the positive acceptance of difference while being "different" is incompatible with the established cultural assumptions of elementary schools. Most teachers and parents perceived their role in integration to be to assimilate students with a visual impairment and "make them like the others." The understandings associated with being different and the contradictions evident as adults and children spoke about this are illustrated in the following excerpts:

[Excerpt 1]

I: *What do Lisa's teachers do which contribute to or detract from her acceptance by peers?*

R: *To contribute to, um..they, I think they tend to involve her as much as they can, not to make her feel left out..the detraction I think would be..her sometimes being singled out, her desk having to be moved closer to the board..which are all things that I know cannot be helped.*

> *And like David [the itinerant teacher] said today about her having to use large print books, you know, they are things which do tend to make other kids more aware of her problem. But which by rights there's really no other way to get around it. Her desk has to be moved up a little bit closer to the board, her printing has to be..reading has to be enlarged, and it's unfair but does tend to single her out and point to her disability more, you know. And I don't think there will ever be any way around that. [parent]*

[Excerpt 2]

I: *What do you see as the teacher's role in the social integration of a student with a visual impairment?*

R: *..Well, I think one role is to, more or less try and treat him or her just like everybody else. Because I think the more exceptions you make..the differences are emphasized with kids. So I think it's best to just treat everybody the same.*

I: *Umm.*

R: *..I think you have to give, I think you have to be prepared to, to do some extra helping and so on..I think the most important part is more or less, treat everybody the same. [teacher]*

As can be seen in the above excerpts, a conflict exists between both wanting the child not to be treated as different, yet having to treat the child differently, and in doing this, feeling "badly" about it. In this study there was no evidence of unconditional acceptance of students or of being different as a positive attribute of a student. The positive acceptance of difference was neither routinely promoted nor enhanced in the elementary classrooms observed. In fact, being different was synonymous with being a "misfit."

Children with a visual impairment cannot escape their "differentness" nor can those who are physically or mentally disabled. Successful social integration assumes a climate of positive acceptance of difference which was not prevalent in the schools in this study. Parents and educators must recognize that these differences exist and work to find adaptations which accommodate learning objectives without devaluing students because they may be different. In fact, a key tenet of teaching is to attend to "individual differences" in instruction and to maximize learning by building on a student's identified learning strengths. Unfortunately, child-centred instruction was a sporadic practice in all but one of the classrooms observed.

The differentness of students with a visual impairment challenged the basic assumptions of the existing school culture both in the classroom and on the playground. The differences in some of their social, cognitive, and physical development needs were incompatible with the basic assumptions of school culture relevant to such things as the way teachers teach and the negotiated rules of group affiliation for students.

The second contradiction prominent during the study was associated with the fact that the goals of integration were incongruent with the predominately competitive learning environment of classrooms. Therefore, the second contradiction was between the stated intention of the student with a visual impairment to be able to progress at her/his own rate following an individualized education program, and the pressure to compete for recognition which was primarily available to those who performed "the best", regardless of the activity. In the elementary classrooms in this study, students struggled to be first—academically, athletically, and socially. They were rewarded with stickers for reading the most books, by having their project chosen to be displayed or to go on to the provincial contest, by being assigned to be first in line, and, in short, for being the smartest, fastest, neatest, quietest, that is, "the best." These things were valued. Therefore, acknowledgement of accomplishments resulting from concerted efforts, that is, being the best you could be, was definitely insignificant in comparison to being "the best" in the class. Possible alternatives to this scenario will be discussed in Chapter 7.

In the following excerpts the manner in which competition pervades the elementary school environment and the frustrations it creates for those who are not the top performers are apparent:

> [Excerpt 1]
> The students work away until it is almost time for gym. Mr. Coates hands out the spelling test from a previous week. He says, "Some of you did very well. A lot of the marks were in the 80s and 90s." He calls out the marks of those in this range as he gives them to each student. Children who did not score in this range are given their test without having their marks announced. They sit silently with their eyes glued to their desks. The children with marks over 80 hold up their papers and exchange information about their grades with the other children who have done well. [observation notes]

> [Excerpt 2]
> I: *What are the advantages and disadvantages, for parents, of having a child with a visual impairment integrated in a regular classroom?*
> R: *The advantage, would be that they are being treated the same as other kids. You hope they are anyway. That they're being taught to realize, you know, that this is just an everyday thing. It is not a real problem, that you don't have to be with a special school or a special this or that just because of your vision. Disadvantage ..that sometimes your child is not going to measure up to the other kids in the class. That the teacher will give them, you know, the benefit of the doubt and say the reason the printing is not as good is because she's visually impaired. You know, like, there was a time I even said to Mrs. Briggs and David [itinerant teacher], I said, "Why can't she get an 'A'?" You know, I said, "If she's doing her absolute best, why can't she get an 'A'?" Will she never in her lifetime get an "A"? Because you know, even her "B" is still not as good as some kids' work. But I said, "Why, if she's doing her*

absolute best?" And she did get an "A" second term, in a couple of things.

I: *She did.*

R: *Yeah, but I, you know, felt looking at her work..I thought it's just as good or she tried just as hard as so and so did. You know? [parent]*

[Excerpt 3]

I: *Have you noticed other children in your class who seem to feel left out?*

R: *Sometimes I think there's some people.*

I: *Who would you say?*

R: *Sometimes, I think that Joanne feels left out if she did something wrong and she's asked to maybe go to a lower group. Just today, she got brought down to the lowest group [in math] and she felt bad because she liked the group she was in cuz most of her friends were in it.*

I: *What group was she in?*

R: *A, no B.*

I: *Have you noticed any other kids who seem to feel left out in your class?*

R: *Justin..I think he feels left out because he has to go, to go to a Special Ed class and he probably feels left out because he can't be in our class in the morning, just cause he knows that he can't do something that we're doing. [Grade 6 classmate]*

[Excerpt 4]

[We have been talking about extra-curricular activities designed specifically for those with a visual impairment in which Charles might be involved. His mother has explained their schedule hasn't allowed Charles' participation this fall.]

I: *Do you have objections to activities that are just for those who are visually impaired?*

R: *No! No! No, I realize Charles needs to be around other kids with visual impairments, too. And I would like to get him into something like that, where he just doesn't have to compete. And, you know, work ten times as hard all the time, but ah, maybe, after Christmas we'll be able to fit it in. [parent]*

For integrated students with a visual impairment, excessively competitive classrooms were hostile social environments. Their responses, when they were visually unable to meet the challenges, varied: Peter initiated conversations extolling those things in which he excelled; Lisa defiantly refused to participate and either put her head down or did something else; Tony persevered regardless of the task; Jamie sat out waiting patiently for the activity to change; and Charles hung his head and seemed very morose. Regardless of their response, all of these children frequently perceived specific situations to be hopeless — because of their visual impairment they were unable to compete. Knowing they could not do well, they frequently did not participate.

Integration assumes the presence of individualized programming and instruction, that is, it assumes attention will be given to the different learning styles, strengths and needs of students as they are taught. In this study, teachers were observed to teach primarily to the class as a whole. Individualized instruction, that is, instruction modified to address a student's higher and/or lower level of performance or to make effective use of learning strengths, was a rare occurrence during the five months of observation. While some principals and teachers spoke of the need to adapt programs and assist students to learn at their own rate, in practice, programs were rarely adapted and all children in most classes were expected to be doing exactly the same thing and using exactly the same learning materials. That is, they were not expected to be different. Therefore, the need for individualized programming or modified instructional techniques by a student with a visual impairment was incompatible with the basic approach to learning and the somewhat competitive nature of elementary schools observed in this study.

Sapon-Shevin (1978) suggested the existence of these contradictions associated with both competition and the positive acceptance of difference almost two decades ago:

> *If we, as educators and as a society, have a responsibility for insuring the success of all children in schools, then we cannot also perpetuate a system that creates deviants and failures by its competitive teaching and evaluation system. The issue of competition is closely related to how differences are viewed. Schools transmit a mixed message with regard to differences: 1) You must all be alike (the value of conformity). 2) You must be better than everyone else (competition). When examined more closely, however, these messages are not at all contradictory, but are indicative of the fact that differences per se are not esteemed and that students are likely to be judged along a single continuum. In school, students are sorted out along the same continuum, but along that continuum those differences that lead to a better performance are rewarded. (p. 120)*

Clearly, these contradictions are still present in elementary schools years after the introduction of integration.

The Dilemmas

As children with a visual impairment have been integrated they have challenged the beliefs, values, and assumptions of the predominant cultures, that of teachers and pupils. This challenge has produced dilemmas associated with the social acceptance and interaction of integrated students. A dilemma is created when people are forced to choose between two alternatives, each alternative having negative consequences. Several were evident in this study;

six are discussed in this section. These six dilemmas were associated with the following:

- the use of adaptive equipment, materials and teaching strategies
- the types of adaptive behaviours developed by students with a visual impairment
- the degree of openness surrounding the discussion of visual impairment
- the relationship between program adaptations and inclusion of the student with a visual impairment
- the accessibility of friendship to students with a visual impairment
- the pressures and responsibilities expected of teachers.

Use of adaptive equipment

The first dilemma is associated with the use of adaptive aids. In an attempt to compensate for a reduction in or lack of vision and, hence, restrictions on access to visual information required to successfully complete routine daily tasks, adaptive equipment (e.g., computers, braille writers, talking calculators or those with large print displays), materials (e.g., tactile maps, large print books) and teaching strategies (e.g., hand-over-hand demonstrations, verbalization of words as they are written on the board) have been developed. In many cases these have been designed specifically for students with a visual impairment and acknowledged as distinctive components required for effective educational programs for this population.

When introduced to the regular public school classroom, these adaptations, while promoting the independence of the student with a visual impairment, frequently interfere with social interaction and acceptance. For example, Tony, the boy who was totally blind, had to move to a working area adjacent to his group to complete all written tasks because his braille writer and print transcriber could not physically be accommodated on his desk located with the other three group members. Charles, a boy with low vision, sat alone at a large desk designed for two students because his large print books and materials required so much desk space. His classmates were seated in pairs with their single sized desks pushed together. As well, dilemmas were created in relation to the provision of help by classmates. Before Tony was able to independently make his way throughout the school, students were assigned or volunteered to take him. Much social interaction, (e.g., laughter, joking, pushing and shoving) characterized these excursions. Once Tony had mastered independent travel using his cane he had to manoeuvre alone and classmates were requested to avoid speaking with him while he was using his cane since, for safety reasons, his full attention was to be focused on moving carefully within his environment. One itinerant teacher describes this dilemma as follows:

R: *I've also found that sometimes kids that accept the use of the aids and what not, are those that have the most difficult time socially. Whereas, those that have almost rejected using the aids are accepted socially. So it's a trade off between..social acceptance and independence and academic success, sometimes.*

I: *So whenever you intervene to assist the person to perform at a level of independence similar to that of their peers, at the same time you add..[interrupts]*

R: *You're adding..I find the students that are, right through to high school, and I've just noticed this in the last few years, those that are most adept at using all these aids, you know, be it white cane, telescopic aids, CCTV's, braille writers, whatever. The kids that want them and are very adept at using them, are less socially accepted than the kids that aren't. Because the kids that don't use them depend on the other students. And often times the other students like to lend a helping hand and that way the..bond develops..and even now, for instance the white cane, you know, as much as we promote it, ah, once a white cane goes down the hallway, everyone disperses and the blind student doesn't, isn't any longer in touch with other students. Even the way a normally sighted student would bump into another in the hall, the student with a white cane misses this.*

I: *Umhmm.*

R: *So they lose that, even that physical contact. So it's, you know, often what, I've found, there is a definite dilemma. [itinerant teacher]*

Thus, for the integrated child with a visual impairment dilemmas related to their social interaction were created both when receiving help or when using aids which permitted independent performance of a task. If the child accepted assistance he/she was often perceived to be less competent or more dependent than classmates but opportunities for positive social interaction were enhanced when working with a buddy. Similarly, when the student with a visual impairment had mastered the use of adaptive aids, thus enhancing independent performance, the use of such aids was often either incompatible with social interaction or limited the opportunity for such.

Adaptive Behaviours Developed by Students

A second kind of dilemma was associated with the adaptive behaviours developed by students with a visual impairment to compensate for their vision loss. For example, all four children with low vision had large handwriting which was frequently difficult to decipher. Although exchanging scribblers to correct or edit each other's work was a common practice in the elementary classrooms observed, few classmates appeared receptive to the sometimes onerous task of deciphering the handwriting of the student with a visual impairment. As well, the student with a visual impairment often has difficulty deciphering the cursive writing of classmates. The solution was usually to have the teacher correct the work of the student with a visual impairment and then have her/him listen while classmates corrected one another's work. Also, the close reading distance required by children with a visual impairment frequently interfered with the sharing of worksheets or project material during group assignments.

One of the more vivid examples of a dilemma created between an effective functional adaptation developed by a student with a visual impairment and its effect upon classmates is illustrated in the following excerpt from the researcher's observation notes.

> It is recess. Just after Tony leaves the school he reaches out and takes hold of a small boy from another class who walks with him to the equipment area. They walk with their arms around each other's shoulders. When they get to the equipment area he leaves Tony. Tony is alone momentarily and as a boy passes by, Tony reaches out and grabs him, holding on to his arm. They walk with their arms around each other's shoulders talking as they go. When they stop Tony takes his arm off his shoulder and grabs on to one of a group of four boys running by. He holds on to the backs of their jackets as they run and they laugh and wrestle. The boys run off leaving Tony alone again. He waits for a few seconds and then reaches out and grabs a girl who is going by. Next, three girls surround him and he tries to catch them. They chant, "Tony can't catch me." He waits until they get quite close then grabs one. One little girl slips out of her jacket to escape and he cheers, "I've got a jacket!" As they are playing Tony's sneaker lace is untied and one of the girls kneels down and ties it for him. A few minutes later she ties his other sneaker. He seems to be enjoying this game and the three continue to play or taunt him until the bell rings. The three girls with whom he is playing are not in his class but seem to be about the same age. They run for the school leaving Tony alone. Just as Tony reaches out to grab a passer-by, a teacher asks a girl to take Tony to the line up. She takes him to the back of the line and Debbie [a girl from his class] takes his hand and takes him to the front of the line. He enters the school first although many children have been lined up before him.

Tony's functional adaptation, that is, reaching out and grabbing a passerby, although often effective in initiating contact with other children, did not always result in positive interaction. Some children, particularly those who did not know Tony well, often objected to his rather unconventional approach to initiating interaction. Yet, given the situation facing him on the noisy, congested playground and the observed tendency of his classmates to avoid him, his strategy did ensure interaction. For Tony, this was a dilemma he faced daily.

Open Discussion of Visual Impairment

A third dilemma was associated with the need to discuss visual impairment openly to ensure awareness of the specific implications of a given child's impairment and the belief that such discussion would stigmatize this child. With the exception of the site where the child was totally blind, the term "visually impaired" was not used. Furthermore, there was no evidence of children having discussed what it meant to be visually impaired or how the child with a visual impairment accommodated the visual loss:

> **R**: *Unless the child's having a real problem with it [visual impairment], I don't really..personally I just don't feel it should be really brought out and made a special case, unless you really are a special case, sort of thing. I mean, I know Lisa has a visual impairment, but for as long as she can be very accepted by the school, I think that, that's probably the best [best not to mention the visual impairment]. There are probably things that could be done to make everybody else more aware, but somehow, I have a feeling that when you're made more aware, then the person becomes more different. And someone that's talked about..and that might make it even harder, instead of easier. [classroom teacher]*

Parents also struggled with this dilemma, as is evident in the following excerpt:

> **R**: *I don't think at the beginning of the year they need to say you have a child with a visual impairment in your class and we need to be, you know, be careful of where we leave things, and stuff like that. You know, if she trips over it, so what, I don't think it would be that much of an incident that would, you know, like be a really serious accident or something. Ah, and that way I don't think the classmates would feel as concerned about it. Because I think they ask a lot more questions and they're so accepting of people anyway, that I don't think they need to even be made aware of it. It is good for them to know about it just the same. It's, you know, it's hard to say either way. Because that way they know that Lisa is different, they know that she's visually impaired, but at the same time I don't like it being my child that's being singled out. [parent]*

As mentioned previously, this reluctance by teachers and parents to even mention "visual impairment" was perceived by both the students with a visual impairment and their classmates to imply visual impairment was a "bad thing." Frequently the child's visual impairment was perceived by many peers and the students with a visual impairment alike, as something for which one should be ashamed. For adults, there seemed to be a belief that if people were uninformed about the impairment they would not treat the child as if he/she was impaired, that is, "different":

> **R**: *A lot of people and a lot of teachers in this school aren't even aware that Jamie has a handicap. And I think probably, ah, if they're not aware he has a handicap then, they just treat him like any other kid. [classroom teacher]*

Thus, the benefits of greater knowledge and increased insight in relation to visual impairment were frequently overlooked so as to avoid calling attention to the child's visual disability. In a social environment which did not promote the positive acceptance of difference, open discussions of visual impairment created a dilemma. As well, it is clear that the absence of discussion relevant to the child's disability could be seen to contribute to the classmates' persistently wrong information about the implications of vision loss (e.g., difficulty with making eye contact, limitations with regard to some types of activities but not others).

Limited Adaptation of Instruction or Programs

A fourth dilemma, closely related to the third, was associated with the reluctance of teachers to adapt programs or activities to enhance the participation of the student with a visual impairment because they felt they were treating the student differently by doing so. Teachers routinely presented lessons without adaptations or accommodations which would either provide access or enhance the ease of access to the information for the visually impaired. Some explained this practice as a purposeful strategy to avoid emphasizing the child's visual impairment or making the student "stand out" as different; others perceived the necessary adaptation to detract from the learning of classmates; and others, unfortunately, perceived themselves to have limitations upon their time and/or skill. Thus, there was a dilemma created between the need for adaptations to access the information being taught and the teacher's reluctance to acknowledge the child's visual impairment by making adaptations. Teachers who perceived overt adaptations as emphasizing the child's disability or accentuating her/his differences in comparison to classmates, seemed to be most uncomfortable with the integration process and seemed to have limited insight into its purpose. An extreme example of this dilemma was the routine distribution of a picture book used in French lessons to the child who was totally blind. His teacher felt she was contributing to his ability to do "exactly the same as the other children" by having him hold the print text being used by his classmates.

Skrtic (1987) believed that school programs are "the product of a particular knowledge tradition that is based on the customs and conventions of a professional subculture [educators]" (p. 21). This results in the teacher addressing only the identified student needs which are compatible with those programs or services he/she has to offer. Therefore, this:

> *is not a problem as long as the student's needs actually match what the professional has to offer, but when the learning style and individual needs of a particular student do not match the professional's repertoire of standard programs the student gets forced artificially into one program or another or forced out of the system altogether. (Skrtic, 1987, p. 21)*

For integrated students with a visual impairment in this study, their social, academic and physical development needs were frequently unique to or incompatible with existing programs, and thus, poorly accommodated.

Unfortunately, for the students with a visual impairment this dilemma had three potentially negative consequences. First, they did not receive the assistance or information which would enhance their performance and possibly improve perceptions related to their competence level — both their own and their peers. Second, the teacher's actions, perceived to be one of ignoring the child's visual impairment, had an implicit, negative message regarding the importance of the child with a visual impairment as a valued student in the regular classroom. Finally, when the child with a visual impairment was treated exactly as classmates, for example, given visual materials when tactile materials were required, confusion was created for students who were uncertain about the abilities and limitations associated with this child, as well as how to appropriately accommodate a student with a visual impairment. This may have contributed to the existence of some of the inaccurate expectations routinely observed during observation.

Accessibility of Friendship

A fifth dilemma facing students with a visual impairment was related to the children who were willing to associate with them on the playground. None of the students with a visual impairment in this study routinely interacted with either the popular group from their class or with a group typical of other children of the same gender at their grade level. It appeared the common factor bringing together the child with a visual impairment and her/his playmate on the playground was the desire to have someone with whom to play. However, as mentioned earlier, children acquired a reputation based on their association and routine interaction with an inappropriate playmate. The frequent interaction between the student with a visual impairment and unpopular peers did little to enhance the social acceptance and interaction of integrated students.

Parents struggled with the dilemma of whether to discourage their child's association with children they perceived to be undesirable playmates or to promote any form of companionship. Frequently the only "friend" their child seemed to have was an unpopular classmate. The following excerpt illustrates one parent's perception of this issue:

I: *What's your feeling about his friendship with Justin?*
R: *..Oh! This is confidential, right?*
I: *Yes.*
R: *Well, Justin's sort of..he's an odd kid. He's different. [Long pause] I don't think he's a friend that I would want Charles to have for life. I'd like to have Charles to have a more out-going friend that could help Charles more. You know what I'm saying?*
I: *Umm.*

R: *Yeah, you know, somebody that could..Charles needs.. well..he needs somebody to, he needs a friend that would accept him for what he is but then, be good for him too.*
I: *Umhmm.*
R: *Yeah. I don't think Justin's good for Charles.*
I: *What types of..when you say he's not good for Charles, what are the types of things you find don't seem to be good for Charles?*
R: *Well..he's not mature. Charles needs somebody more mature. Like, I think Charles is more mature, a lot more mature than Justin.*
I: *Yeah, he needs some..that's one of the things that I would, you know, I would like for Charles, is to have a friend, sort of a friend that he could call and, well, I guess that comes later on, doesn't it? When they get older. [parent]*

Therefore, for students with a visual impairment, there was often a dilemma created in choosing between being alone on the playground or associating with an unpopular classmate.

Teacher Pressures and Responsibilities

A final dilemma routinely arose in relation to how the teacher responded to the student with a visual impairment in the classroom. The elementary school day is highly structured in terms of time. There are designated periods and amounts of time scheduled to collect milk money, go to other classes (e.g., French, physical education, music), go out for recess, eat lunch, etc. Teachers and students were frequently rushing to meet these time limits. However, four of the students who were visually impaired routinely required additional time to complete most activities, including independently taking out and putting away books and materials. Teachers were often faced with the dilemma of doing something for the child with a visual impairment or letting her/him complete it despite the delays it entailed for the entire class.

For the student with a visual impairment the dilemma was often a choice among being perceived as incapable of completing an assignment if the teacher helped, taking it home to finish it for homework, or being blamed for slowing down the entire class. When teachers did things for the child with a visual impairment in order to "pick up the pace" or meet a time limit, classmates frequently perceived the child with a visual impairment to be receiving special attention, extra help or to be less competent as a student. In the final analysis, the integration of a child with a visual impairment in the regular classroom created many complex situations and dilemmas which were pervasive and difficult to address or overcome given the present structure of elementary schools.

The Implications for Evolving Self-Concept

As contradictions and dilemmas were identified in this study, so were the potential implications for the student with a visual impairment. Perhaps the most significant of these was the risk to the development of a positive self-concept and to high self-esteem. As people respond to their environment in terms of the meanings they construct, the process of social interaction is the source of their developing perceptions. The self is given meaning through the process of interaction as a result of the attitudes expressed by significant others toward it. Therefore, one's self-concept develops in relation to the meanings others construct and reflect toward one, both explicitly and implicitly, during social interaction.

In this study the children who were visually impaired ranged from six to almost thirteen years of age. Despite their varying levels of maturity, visual disability, age, and social skills, they had learned some common beliefs relevant to visual impairment and those who were visually impaired. These beliefs, identified during the analysis of data, are as follows:

- People who are visually impaired must depend upon sighted people for help.
- People who are visually impaired need more help to do most things than do sighted people.
- Sighted people can do more things than people who are visually impaired can.
- Sighted people can do most things better than people who are visually impaired can.
- Sighted people are thankful they are not visually impaired.
- People who are visually impaired are different, and hence inferior to sighted people.
- Sighted people think they are superior to people who are visually impaired.
- Sighted people think people who are visually impaired are not as intelligent as they are.
- Being visually impaired causes extra problems for parents and teachers.
- Parents wish their children were not visually impaired.
- Sighted children prefer to play with other sighted children.
- Children with a visual impairment are less desirable as "best friends" than are those who are fully sighted.

As the self-concepts of these children were gradually evolving during the process of interaction, these beliefs were prominent features in their daily environments. Since "the perceptions and feelings an individual has about the self, whether realistic or not, cumulatively mold and shape the self-concept" (Tuttle, 1984, p. 63), the potential for students with a visual impairment in this study to construct positive self-concepts was at risk.

Self-esteem, the evaluative component of self-concept, involves comparing one's performance with a standard which is either set by others or by oneself (Tuttle, 1984). In this study, the performance of the four students with low vision, both in school and on the playground, was routinely viewed by themselves and their peers to be inferior to that of other children. In many ways, the child who was totally blind had a reprieve from the frequency and severity of comparisons experienced by children with low vision. He could not compare his braille to the printed work of his classmates, nor could they judge the quality of his work in comparison to their own. Thus, spontaneous comments concerning his level of performance were far less frequent than those for students with low vision. This boy was the only one of the five students with a visual impairment who perceived being visually impaired as something which would attract friends, as a reason other children might like to play with him.

For these children, being visually impaired was a predominant aspect of their being. During their school life, there seemed to be rarely an activity where some compensatory skill or accommodating action was not required if they were to actively participate with their peers. When things did not go well, it was because they were visually impaired. When their peers excluded them, it was because they were visually impaired. When they were slow to finish their work, it was because they were visually impaired. They seemed to perceive their level of control over the course of their own actions as being significantly restricted by their visual impairment. For students with a visual impairment there is an inherent danger that their less than desirable level of acceptance by and interaction with peers be perceived as an inevitable consequence of being visually impaired. Given such a perception, "normal" social interactions with those who are sighted might seem to be a rather hopeless aspiration.

The vulnerability of students with a visual impairment, in regard to their exclusion by peers, seemed to increase with age and grade level. As children progressed through school, groups appeared to become more exclusive. At the same time, the level of competence required to participate in most activities increased. For example, by grade six, boys were expected to be skilled ball players and the difficulties experienced by the student with a visual impairment were blatant by contrast. As well, in the classroom the quantity and rate of reading and writing assignments had significantly increased for students by the late elementary school grades. However, the reading and writing rates of the students with a visual impairment had not increased proportionately.

These observations seem to support the conclusions of Goupil and Comeau (1983) and Eaglestein (1975) who found students with a visual impairment to become less accepted by peers the longer they had been integrated. Friendships mature and children who are excluded in the early years of school have difficulty being accepted because they have not been exposed to the maturing or evolving process and its experiences. Children who are unpopular seem to become more unpopular with age as their reputation for being unpopular becomes better established. Obviously, the provision of programs to promote the social acceptance of all children who are at risk of being excluded by the majority of their peers is crucial.

Conclusion

This research has contributed to a more comprehensive understanding of the issues intrinsic to the acceptance and interaction of students with a visual impairment who are integrated in regular classrooms. It has revealed the complexity of the integration process and the need for educators to attend to the total social environment of schools as students are integrated; some potential starting points by which to address those aspects of school culture which detract from and those which encourage the successful social integration of visually impaired students; and, more importantly, why it is critical that educators do this.

Research is an evolving process. As insights are developed new perspectives and procedures are also required. There is much that society in general, and educators in particular, have to learn and understand about the social, instructional, and temporal integration of children with disabilities. Current research on integration supports the conclusion that integration is a complex innovation which requires major restructuring of "general education" if the inherent benefits of this process are to be realized. Until both the implicit and explicit issues relevant to the integration of students with a visual impairment can be acknowledged and addressed, these students will continue to encounter a less than positive social environment in which to spend their school days.

This does not imply a return to segregated educational placements for these children. To do so would be to abandon the opportunity to change those aspects of the public school system which interfere with the full integration of those with disabilities and which are also barriers to the successful performance and affective development of many other students considered "at risk" in our schools (e.g., unpopular and rejected children). Indeed, it is the professional responsibility of educators to make a commitment to promote the social, physical, and cognitive development of all children.

In the next section, guidelines and suggestions to promote the social acceptance and interaction of students with a visual impairment will be presented. As is obvious from the research reported in previous chapters, planning will be necessary at the school level to incorporate the specific aspects of programs designed to address the identified needs in any given situation.

Section III

Promoting Social Integration in our Schools

7

Enhancing Social Acceptance and Interaction: Where to Begin?

Introduction

It is evident that educators are being asked to accommodate a more diverse student population in the regular classroom than has been the case in the past. Furthermore, teachers are routinely being expected to assist with children experiencing a multiplicity of social problems (e.g., child abuse, disruptive family situations). Obviously, the need to attend to the social/emotional development of students, their level of self-esteem, and the social skills required to succeed in our society is common to all children, including those who have a visual impairment. The critical importance of affective education, given the nature of today's society and the problems its children encounter, can no longer be denied.

In this chapter guidelines and suggestions to enhance the social acceptance and interaction of children with a visual impairment are presented. Considerations specific to school programming, students with a visual impairment, and classmates of these students are outlined. This is followed by the presentation of an array of suggestions for teachers and parents. In the social environment of the school these considerations and suggestions are interrelated and frequently interdependent. Formal intervention must take a broad perspective encompassing the multiplicity of variables and input from all participants—administrators, teachers, parents, and students. It is also important to consider that the actions taken to establish a social environment that will enhance the social integration of students with a visual impairment will simultaneously have a positive effect upon the affective development of all students in the school.

School Level Considerations

The integration of students with a visual impairment should be perceived as a significant educational innovation requiring a formal plan for implementation. This plan must include such things as training and inservice opportunities for classroom teachers, identification of school philosophies and practices, preparation of the student population, procedural guidelines, monitoring and evaluation procedures, and adequate funding for essential resources. Of critical importance is the leadership essential to address and manage the cultural changes integration entails.

School Philosophies and Practices

As discussed in Chapter 4, the basic cultural assumptions of any organization are the underlying and unconscious beliefs which have come to be taken for granted as intrinsic to the organization and thereby, guide the behaviour of its members (Schein, 1985). Therefore, educators and parents must identify those principles which will be reflected in the social environment of their schools. Discipline, respect for teachers, and an emphasis on academic achievement are common goals of most schools. If the social integration of students with a visual impairment is to be successful, additional principles must be adopted and promoted by school participants. Of particular importance is an emphasis on the affective development of students, the enhancement of high self-esteem, and the need to create a social environment which promotes the positive acceptance of difference and eradicates the stigma associated with being different.

Educators and parents need a risk-free opportunity to explore and discuss their feelings and beliefs relevant to visual impairment. These must be examined to correct misconceptions, to identify prejudices, and to understand how beliefs may influence ones actions in certain situations (e.g., holding lower expectations for students with a visual impairment).

Because teachers have considerable autonomy within their given classrooms, it is critical that staff as a group reach a consensus on philosophies and practice which should guide their work as teachers. These decisions must by made at the school level, not imposed by outside administrators. Such decisions will increase the probability of obtaining active participation and commitment from all educators in the school. As well, there are other employees who need to be aware of the practices being promoted by educators and parents. For example, playground supervisors must be aware of efforts to involve all students in playground activities, including those with a visual impairment. Bus drivers, secretaries, and janitors alike, need to be aware of the beliefs and behaviours which are being nurtured in their school. A consistent philosophy and practices for all adults is a high priority in supportive school environments.

Junior and senior high school educators often focus their attention on course content, viewing the affective components of education to be beyond their responsibility. In the face of recent educational research expounding the critical importance of enhancing the self-esteem of teenagers and preparing youth to deal with the many stresses inherent in living in present day society, effective teachers must establish a balance in their curriculum between process and content and between cognitive and affective domains. The current stay-in-school initiatives evolving across the country are calling for a wholesale restructuring of the education system with a focus on the individual needs of "at-risk" students. In school districts where educators have demonstrated some success in decreasing the dropout rates in high schools, two critical program components have been identified. First, there has been an emphasis on promoting an improvement in self-esteem. Second, the school staff have employed a team approach to program planning for "at-risk" students. Obviously, these two components must become incorporated in any school's philosophy before they can be reflected in school practices.

The Collaborative Team

Schools need to form collaborative teams committed to enhancing the social acceptance and positive interaction of students with a visual impairment. Team membership should include the principal, classroom teachers, teacher of the visually impaired, and parents of the student. The team should also encourage participation from resource personnel such as resource room teachers, guidance counsellors, and school psychologists. In many cases students with a visual impairment and their classmates should be included as contributing members of the team. Teachers who may be involved with the student in future years should also be encouraged to participate on the team. All teachers usually have several students in any given class who struggle with peer acceptance. The presence of a school team committed to the goal of social integration will elicit interest and spontaneous discussion of effective practices or potential ideas. Guided by a principal who routinely espouses the importance of social integration, school staff will be encouraged to attend to social integration in their classrooms.

Planning for social integration requires educators and parents to do just that —have a plan. Each team participant brings a different perspective and, in many cases, different skills and understanding to the team. Since regular classroom teachers have been designated as having the major educational responsibility for students who are integrated in the regular classroom, they should participate fully in the designing of programs and in the implementation of plans. Teachers should also be expected to play an active part in the ongoing decision making involved in the placement and programming for the students with disabilities in their classrooms. Parents know their child intimately and can work to ensure programming plans address the concerns they consider a priority in relation to the social/emotional development of their child. The teacher of the visually impaired has an in-depth understanding of the implications of vision loss on learning and can help to ensure teaching strategies and materials are appropriate for the particular student. In the final analysis, what is critical to the team is a collaborative approach in which the contribution of each participant is equally valued and the focus of the group is on enhancing the social acceptance and interaction of the student who has a visual impairment.

A Problem-solving Perspective

Social acceptance is a multifaceted phenomenon. There are conceivably hundreds of aspects of a given situation which influence the quantity and quality of social interaction that students with a visual impairment will experience. While there are some teaching strategies and learning environments which are commonly believed to enhance or detract from social acceptance, many variables are unique to specific students and particular situations. Therefore, educators and parents need to develop a "problem-solving perspective" as they analyze and assess intervention in a given situation. What activities are increasing interaction? Is this interaction resulting in positive or negative experiences for the student with a visual impairment and for classmates? What could be done to increase the opportunities available for the student with a visual impairment to reciprocate the help received from classmates? While identical questions might be posed in two different schools, the responses may vary significantly. Approaches developed at a given school by educators and parents who are aware of their unique circumstances and those of their students will be the most successful.

Observation is an invaluable source of information. It can help to identify teaching strategies and social environments which enhance and detract from social acceptance and interaction for a specific student in a given setting. Observation data collected by various members of the team in a variety of in-class and outside-class situations and at different times during the school year provide the basis for effective intervention.

Gathering information to use for both planning and decision making should not be restricted to the adults in the school. Generating solutions to identified problems may often include students who are visually impaired and their classmates. Their perceptions often provide adults with valuable insight into the situations they encounter and, thus, potential solutions to problems.

The dilemmas which arise in relation to the integration of students who are visually impaired (e.g., use of equipment that isolates the student but provides independence) are complex ones. A problem-solving approach can generate appropriate or workable solutions to most of these dilemmas. As strategies or solutions are adopted, all others in the school affected by such decisions must be informed. This increases the likelihood of consistent responses to many of the situations which arise during routine daily activities as well as the understanding of all staff.

Working as a member of a school team, employing a problem-solving perspective, attending meetings, and observing students are time consuming activities. The best of teachers' intentions can be sabotaged if plans are not devised to accommodate the additional demands made upon the time available to teachers to complete many of the tasks involved. This is particularly true in the initial stages of program development. Administrators must consider the most effective ways to employ team members, options for accessing assistance for the teacher, and specific plans to ensure teachers do not become overwhelmed by the task at hand. Undoubtedly, the successful integration of a student with a visual impairment will add to the responsibilities, hence the time commitments, of the classroom teacher. Teachers, expected to play a leading role in the integration process, must receive the support and the assistance necessary to develop an inclusive classroom environment.

Training

In Canada, the majority of teachers are middle-aged. When they were involved in their pre-service training, considerable emphasis was being placed on identifying those students who could benefit from special education placement in segregated classrooms as opposed to strategies to assist such students in the regular classroom. Adaptive teaching methods and materials were considered the domain of special educators—those providing special education services to students enrolled in special education classes or in resource rooms. The integration of students with disabilities has placed the responsibility for instruction with classroom teachers. Unfortunately, teachers are frequently assigned students with special needs regardless of their qualifications or their willingness to pursue additional training.

The professional development of educators is obviously an ongoing process. Every year the education profession is inundated with revised curricula, innovative instructional approaches, and new knowledge relevant to how children learn and develop. As parents and educators in a given school take on the challenge of enhancing the social acceptance of a student with a visual impairment, there are several areas of training which will contribute to the success of their endeavours. They need knowledge and insight relevant to such things as the following:

- the complex philosophical, moral, and pragmatic issues inherent to integration
- knowledge about the nature and implications of visual impairment
- awareness of the social world of children, their perspectives, and the role friendship plays in the affective development of students
- understanding of the rules negotiated by children relevant to acceptance, positive interaction, and friendship
- knowledge of affective education and how to incorporate instruction in the classroom
- familiarity with social skills training methods and concerns and adaptations specific to students with a visual impairment
- awareness of the ongoing process inherent to the development of high self-esteem and the variables which contribute to a sense of selfworth.

These areas of knowledge are not isolated but frequently interrelated in a variety of ways (e.g., active participation with peers is correlated with high self-esteem). Insight into these broad issues will facilitate the incorporation of this knowledge into programs designed to address the social integration of students with a visual impairment.

It is critical that we recognize the need for both parent and teacher education in these identified areas. It cannot be assumed that any member of the collaborative team has had previous access to this knowledge. In their pre-service training, teachers of the visually impaired are rarely exposed to aspects of pupil culture in the public school environment or, perhaps, even specific training to enhance social acceptance. Methodology relevant to affective education is not a compulsory course in most education programs. Parents will also bring a range of knowledge relevant to parenting and child development. What is essential is that members of the collaborative team understand the issues involved in social integration and how to implement and evaluate programs which will enhance the affective development of students. Obviously, there must be flexibility to experiment with a variety of strategies. As well, there must be the support of a collaborative team to evaluate the effectiveness of planned intervention designed to promote both social and instructional integration of students with a visual impairment.

Cooperative Learning

Cooperative learning has been identified as a learning structure which has the potential to enhance the acceptance of students with disabilities who are integrated in the regular classroom (Johnson & Johnson, 1981). It is a process which encompasses such things as cooperation with peers, motivation by peers, shared responsibility for learning goals, understanding of group dynamics, and the learning of essential social skills. It is not the intention of this text to promote the adoption of a specific approach to learning. However, cooperative learning can offer educators effective strategies in their efforts to promote social integration.

Cooperative learning is far more than assigning children to a group to work on a given task. There are five basic elements of cooperative learning — positive interdependence, face to face interaction, individual accountability, interpersonal and small group skills, and group processing (Johnson, Johnson & Holubec, 1990). These are presented and discussed in relation to their potential influence on the social acceptance and interaction of students with a visual impairment.

Positive interdependence is the first prerequisite for a cooperative group and exists when students believe the group cannot be successful unless each member is also successful. Each group member is responsible for both her/his individual learning as well as that of each of the other members of the group. The task for a student with a significant cognitive disability is adjusted to ensure meaningful participation and to prevent this student from being perceived by other members as lowering the chances for the group's success. Positive interdependence promotes the sharing of ideas, responsibilities, materials and resources as well as the active participation of each member of the group. The tendency of capable students to take over and complete most of the work, or for unmotivated students to provide limited input, is eliminated because the group's success is determined by the level of achievement of each member. Thus, each member has a vested interest in the learning of every other student.

When a student with a visual impairment is working in a group characterized by positive interdependence a number of significant opportunities for social integration are inevitable. For example, the student has an opportunity to help other students, make meaningful contributions to the work of the group, be seen by peers to be doing and mastering the same task as other group members, and participate in much social interaction. There are also other positive spin-offs associated with working in a cooperative group. To participate, the student who is visually impaired must have access to the information being learned by the group members. This requires that teachers or members of the group attend to the student's need for access to information and timely explanations of new concepts. Of major significance is the opportunity cooperative learning provides for students with a visual impairment to routinely demonstrate their learning strengths and abilities as they are actively involved in completing the group assignment.

The second element of cooperative learning is face-to-face interaction. This component requires that students promote each other's learning through interaction such as explaining information or encouraging the learning of others. Glasser (1969) has suggested that we learn 10% of what we read, 20% of what we hear, 30% of what we see, 70% of what is discussed with others, and 95% of what we teach someone else. Thus, face-to-face interaction exemplifies a very dynamic method of learning. Group pressure may be exerted to encourage reluctant participants to increase their contributions. Furthermore, through the interaction inherent in this aspect of cooperative learning, the members come to know each other as individuals. They are in a situation where they cannot avoid interaction with a given student but must make considerable efforts to negotiate positive social interaction if the group is to be successful.

As mentioned earlier in the text, face-to-face exchange for students with a visual impairment is typically less frequent than for their classmates, thereby reducing their opportunity to practice and refine social skills. In a cooperative learning group the student with a visual impairment has an opportunity to get to know classmates as well as to obtain a realistic perspective of their own strengths and weaknesses. In turn, classmates have an opportunity to overcome their fears or alter negative attitudes associated with interactions with a student with a visual impairment. For both parties, this happens spontaneously as they become more familiar through routine interaction.

Face-to-face interaction provides a tremendous opportunity for the student who is visually impaired to state and clarify conceptual learning in an accepting environment. Classmates will soon become skilled at detecting misconceptions or misunderstandings which often result when vision loss interferes with access to information. With practice and experience peers become well informed not only of the implications of vision loss on learning but of alternative ways to present information which is more useful for a student with a visual impairment.

Individual accountability is the third element of cooperative learning. Because each group member is responsible for learning the assigned material, the teacher may use individual testing, random questioning, and group self checking to ensure individual accountability. It is difficult for reluctant students to "get by" on the efforts of others. For students with significant learning difficulties, aspects of the individualized education plan can be incorporated within the group assignment and the student can be tested on these aspects. In many integrated placements, reduced expectations for students with a visual impairment are common. With individual accountability only performance differences outlined in the student's individualized education plan will be accommodated. Therefore, the expectations for students with a visual impairment are more apt to be those common to other participants in the group. The students themselves coach and evaluate one another as they strive to ensure each participant has mastered the material assigned. This process in itself creates the expectation that the student who is visually impaired will not only learn but will coach others. Because the teacher provides feedback on both the group's achievements and those of individual members, the classmates of the student who is visually impaired receive accurate information about the performance of this student. Therefore, there are routine opportunities for classmates to receive accurate information about the capabilities of the student with a visual impairment.

Learning and using interpersonal and small group skills is the fourth element of cooperative learning. Teachers provide formal instruction in specific social and organization skills which assist students to get into their groups, organize their environment, and follow interpersonal communication strategies which promote positive interaction and learning. The emphasis is on two categories of skills—those required to work effectively with people and those which facilitate the completion of the task. "People skills" include such things as how to listen effectively, disagree in a nice way, dignify the errors of others, encourage others to speak, reduce group tension, and express appreciation. Examples of "task skills" include staying on task, paraphrasing, seeking opinions, delegation, following directions, and checking the understanding of all members of the group. These collaborative skills are, of course, essential to effective group dynamics at any level — home, school, or work place. In many ways, the degree to which students learn and incorporate these two categories of skills is highly correlated with the success of cooperative learning, in general.

Because the teacher is instructing students in social skills as part of the process of cooperative learning, many of the skills needed by the student with a visual impairment can be addressed naturally in the classroom. Making eye contact when speaking with someone or assessing a person's response to one's idea from facial expressions or the tone of voice are skills which are frequently troublesome for those with a visual impairment. In a classroom incorporating cooperative learning, such skills would be presented and practised as a routine part of the learning process.

In the group setting, a student with a visual impairment has regular opportunities to get to know and trust classmates, encourage and assist others, and resolve conflict in a constructive manner. Practice of such skills dramatically increases both the likelihood of this student interacting in a meaningful way outside the classroom and the probability that educators will address the need for social skills instruction for this student because participation in the group depends upon effective communication skills. Skills which are most problematic for students with a visual impairment become evident when the group members are asked to assess the use of specific skills by group members.

The fifth basic element of cooperative learning is group processing. Group members assess and discuss how well they accomplished the assigned goal and generate strategies to overcome those behaviours or actions which detracted from the degree of success. This debriefing process is a powerful means of having students analyze and learn from their errors as well as providing an opportunity for students to take pride in their accomplishments and have their performance acknowledged.

For the student with a visual impairment, group processing provides an opportunity to share one's perspectives on a given situation with those of classmates. This increases the awareness of both parties. As well, it ensures that students with a visual impairment receive feedback about their performance. Did mannerisms such as rocking interfere with communication? Did the student direct her gaze toward the speaker? Was the student able to encourage and assist other students in learning the material? Were the student's organizational skills, working habits, or pace appropriate? These are the types of interactions which are frequently limited or nonexistent in traditional classrooms where learning is individualistically or competitively structured.

In this brief overview of cooperative learning it is obvious that this learning structure offers both affective and cognitive advantages to students with a visual impairment who are integrated in regular classrooms. It also necessitates teachers learn and refine new interaction skills. Teachers have many responsibilities in orchestrating cooperative learning. They must not only organize the groups and prepare materials but must also structure positive interdependence, accountability and cooperation; explain criteria for success and identified desired behaviours; evaluate the quantity and quality of student learning; and assess group functioning. Cooperative learning requires that students be taught the skills essential to successful learning in groups. It also necessitates that educators learn and become comfortable using a range of instructional practices (e.g., peer editing, open analysis and discussion of relationships, positive acceptance of difference). The learning of skills required to work cooperatively with others will benefit students throughout their lives. In fact, a school staff working cooperatively is the hallmark of an effective school.

For further information on cooperative learning, a list of reference materials is provided in Appendix A.

Assessment and Planning

Before undertaking the intriguing challenge of enhancing the social acceptance and interaction of students with a visual impairment, parents and educators must obtain accurate information upon which to base intervention strategies and plans. A variety of assessment instruments and checklists devised to determine such things as a student's popularity among peers, social skills, and level of self-esteem, as well as the nature of the social environment or school climate can provide essential information for the formulation of plans to enhance social integration. A compilation of appropriate materials is found in Appendix B.

Sociometric scales provide information about children's interpersonal relationships. They attempt to answer questions such as the following: Are individual students liked by most of their peers? How are they perceived by classmates? Which children are most accepting of a particular child? What are the friendship patterns in this classroom? Who identifies a given student as a desired workmate or playmate?

There are three basic types of sociometric techniques. Peer nomination instruments measure children's feelings of friendship toward their peers. Students are asked to name classmates who are their best friends, "okay friends" or not friends. A second technique, referred to as peer rating, provides a general measure of acceptance. With this strategy, children rate each of their classmates on such things as how much they like to work with or play with them. The third sociometric technique is peer observation and involves examining the perceptions of students about their classmates relevant to the student perceived to be the friendliest, best worker, smartest, or most helpful. As might be expected, there are both advantages and disadvantages to the use of the various types of sociometric instruments. For example, some instruments may increase the vulnerability of "at-risk" children if classmates who do not adhere to rules of confidentiality taunt them about being nominated as "not a friend." On the other hand, sociometric techniques are helpful in providing teachers with fairly reliable information about the social status of each of the students in the classroom. As with all assessment tools, the situation and the need for information should guide their use.

An assessment of the student's social skills is a second area where information is essential. A social skills checklist provides an initial overview of the skill strengths and needs of the student and can also be used to record skills which will be taught and mastered during the year. These checklists may be completed by parents, teachers or the students themselves. Typically they include questions about the student's social behaviour, such as whether the student can initiate a conversation, understand the feelings of others, share belongings, or deal appropriately with conflict.

Checklists devised specifically for students with a visual impairment are of tremendous benefit because they incorporate skills which are frequently problematic for those who receive limited visual feedback. The curriculum, *Independent Living* by Loumiet and Levack, 1992 is an excellent example of programming designed specifically for those with a visual impairment. Learning how to compensate for or adapt such skills as directing gaze toward the speaker or refraining from engaging in socially unacceptable mannerisms are critical to programming designed to meet the needs of students with a visual impairment. Because many children with a visual impairment are extremely attentive to auditory information emanating from their environment, it is frequently assumed they will automatically develop skills such as interpreting another's vocal emotion. Research completed by Minter, Hobson, and Pring (1992) has suggested that children with a visual impairment need specific instruction in the accurate interpretation of vocally expressed emotion. Such findings emphasize the importance of comprehensive assessment of each child's skills and abilities prior to initiating the training of social skills.

To illustrate a checklist of skills associated with nonverbal communication developed specifically for individuals with a visual impairment, an excerpt from the *Independent Living* curriculum has been presented in Table 1.

Table 1.

*Social Competence—Nonverbal Communication**

Age	Skills
0-1 Year	1 Use touching to communicate in socially acceptable ways.
2-3 Years	2 Respond appropriately to common auditory signals and/or gestures in familiar contexts. 3 Use a few common gestures to communicate. 4 Refrain from engaging in socially unacceptable mannerisms.
4-7 Years	5 Demonstrate comprehension of common facial expressions in social contexts, and/or use them effectively. 6 Demonstrate comprehension of conventional gestures in social contexts, and/or use them effectively.
8-11 Years	7 Use nonverbal behaviors to indicate interest in a speaker's message. 8 Demonstrate an awareness of socially acceptable and unacceptable body postures and movements in different social situations. 9 Use common forms of body contact to communicate in a conventional manner.

12-15 Years	10 Use a wide variety of nonverbal behaviors to communicate more effectively. 11 Explore ways of obtaining information communicated through nonverbal visual cues. 12 Discuss how cultural differences may affect nonverbal communication, and what the implications of these differences are for social interactions.

[Note: The Independent Living curriculum provides information relevant to each goal on the checklist, sample lesson plans, teaching suggestions, and a wealth of resources and materials.] * Reproduced with permission from Independent Living, Volume I, Social Competence, p. 214, by R. Loumiet and Nvack

If educators and parents are to address the issues related to social integration, the self-esteem of students must be understood and monitored. It is difficult to develop an objective way to measure self-esteem because there is not a standard definition (Chiu, 1992). Questionnaires and checklists completed by the student are the most frequently used type of assessment instrument (e.g., The Piers-Harris Children's Self-Concept Scale). When students have a trusting relationship with the adult administering such tests, responses provide insight into how the students are perceiving their own worth and social behaviour. As with all assessment tools, results should assist educators in developing effective intervention strategies.

Assessment must go beyond the identification of variables relevant to a specific student or the student body in general. Aspects of the social environment and the instructional approaches used by both teachers and parents must be examined in order to address factors which enhance and detract from the social acceptance and interaction of students with a visual impairment. Questions such as the following should be routinely asked in order to assess the school climate: Do teachers accept, practice, and promote the principles of integration? Is the social environment characterized by a sense of respect for students? The ten factors commonly associated with "winning school climates" and examples of each factor are given in Table 2.

Table 2. **The 10 Essentials***

Schools with winning school climates have these 10 factors in common:

1 A supportive, stimulating environment	(e.g., help and support colleagues; champion repect and acceptance)
2 Student-centered	(e.g., include students in decision making; allow for student differences)
3 Positive expectations (e.g., send positive messages; model high standards)	(e.g., send positive messages; model high standards)

4 Feedback	(e.g., send positive messages; model high standards)
5 Rewards	(e.g., catch others succeeding; be candid but positive)
6 A sense of family	(e.g., be involved; acknowledge and deal with conflict)
7 Closeness to parents and community	(e.g., invite feedback; work on consumer satisfaction)
8 Communication	(e.g., be an active listener; keep others informed)
9 Achievement	(e.g., set and track personal, classroom and building level goals; find achievement)
10 Trust	(e.g., be consistent; respect others)

* From *Tips for Improving School Climate* by J.Sweeney

Regardless of the type of instruments being used to collect information for informed decision making, observation will always be a fundamental source of significant information. When considering the social interaction of humans, their unique and often unpredictable behaviours, and the infinite variety of experiences and perspectives one brings to a given situation, observation is sometimes the only procedure which can provide the information or insights needed. Indeed, when examining social integration, observation is mandatory at all levels—assessment, monitoring, and evaluation. It serves two basic functions. First, one is able to experience firsthand the nature of the environment and what is happening. Second, through routine observation one comes to know what to expect in a given environment, the typical and atypical behaviours, and the perceptions of those who routinely participate in the setting.

To master the skills of observation requires training, practice, and refinement. A competent observer can identify what is important and unimportant in a given situation, how people perceive and respond to the actions of others, and aspects that interfere with or contribute to supportive, stimulating school environments. Obviously, effective assessment, monitoring, and programming to enhance social integration requires routine observation by competent observers.

For further information on social skills checklists, sociometric scales, and class climate questionnaires, a list of reference materials is provided in Appendix B.

The Positive Acceptance of Difference

The positive acceptance of difference is a complex concept intrinsically linked with what is valued in our culture. During the early months of a child's first year in school, the importance of conforming to both the teacher's rules and those of the pupil culture are evident to most children. Children are openly rewarded for compliance with these rules through some form of positive reinforcement (e.g., verbal praise) or avoidance of negative consequences (e.g., being reprimanded). Those things which become valued, such as waiting one's turn, doing neat work, or helping a friend on the playground, also become the standard by which individuals are valued. It is ultimately this valuing process which creates the sense of "goodness" or "badness" associated with being different. Along this continuum various degrees of differentness are tolerated depending upon the behaviour or issue being considered. For example, an overweight student who is an invaluable member of the football team may encounter less harassment for his differentness, (i.e. being obese) than will one who does not hold such a position. A gifted child who struggles to comply with organizational rules of the classroom (e.g., attending to the task assigned or placing work in the proper notebook) may be viewed as less different in a classroom where learning through discovery is encouraged than in one in which lessons are presented in a highly structured, teacher dominated manner. In some instances, differentness is dictated by fads or fashions of a given time. Examples include length of hair for boys and shortness of skirts for girls. What is in fashion at one point in time may have negative connotations at another time. As humans we establish norms and values within a given culture which come to be viewed as standards upon which to measure compliance and differentness.

When a student with a visual impairment is enroled in a classroom in the neighbourhood school, there may be a number of differences which immediately distinguish this child from others in the class. As mentioned previously, the student may have learning materials which are different from peers, special equipment which is not used by other students, physical characteristics which are unfamiliar, or unusual behaviours. Furthermore, this student may be provided with assistance to travel outside the classroom, special teachers who visit on a regular basis, or even have an adult assistant assigned to be with her/him for most of the day. Although some of these differences may be eliminated or minimized through thoughtful planning, others are inevitable. We cannot change the differentness imposed by visual impairment. What parents and educators can influence, however, is how difference is valued in our schools and the degree of emphasis placed on acknowledging the similarities.

As educators and parents plan to enhance the social integration of students with a visual impairment, open discussion of what is to be valued in our schools can set the stage for consideration of how best to promote the positive acceptance of difference among children. At the instructional level teachers need to reflect upon such things as evaluating achievement. Is it based upon individual student goals or measured by comparison to the performance of others? How will academic excellence be acknowledged? Which is of greater value, a concerted effort to complete an assignment or the degree of mastery of the assigned material? The approaches associated with various practices send important messages to students relevant to what is or is not valued. Similarly, from an affective education perspective, teachers can emphasize or overlook the importance of understanding others, being sensitive to and valuing differences, and working and playing cooperatively. Just as goals are set for the academic performance of students so must they be outlined for affective development.

The positive acceptance of difference is a value which must be nurtured in our schools. More than any other, it is a prerequisite for the social acceptance of students with a visual impairment. Through both their actions and words, adults send students distinct messages regarding those things or people which are valued by them. Hence, they need to be both aware of the nature of these messages they send and make concerted efforts to model the positive acceptance of difference if their students are to be socialized to perceive this value as an appropriate one.

For further information on school level considerations, a list of reference materials is provided in Appendix D.

Considerations for the Student With a Visual Impairment

A reoccurring theme central to this book is the belief that social integration can only be achieved when all participants in the social environment take responsibility for meeting the many challenges it entails. Although an important component, programs designed to improve the social competence of students with a visual impairment will have limited success if not provided in conjunction with comprehensive programming for classmates, educators and parents. Therefore, as we examine those considerations relevant to students with a visual impairment, it is important to keep in mind the interrelationships these children have with other participants in the social environment of the school in general and the interdependent nature of social acceptance.

Assessment

Assessment is the process of gathering information for the purpose of "(1) specifying and verifying problems and (2) making decisions about students." (Salvia & Ysseldyke, 1991). When planning to enhance the social acceptance and interaction of students with a visual impairment, assessment data is essential to the development of appropriate programming. Formal assessment completed by trained personnel provides information about the child's cognitive abilities, problem solving skills, or level of social cognition. For example, the Wide Range Achievement Test-Revised (WRAT-R) examines the student's auditory processing skills. Such skills are known to play an important role in interpersonal communication. The Piers-Harris Children's Self-Concept Scale provides insight into how students perceive themselves so programming can address the specific needs of the individual. A checklist of social skills help to identify areas of strength and need. As mentioned previously, informal assessment of interaction through observation is often a source of the most valuable information when planning strategies for a particular class or child. Observations should include a variety of settings (e.g., classroom, gym, playground, recreational activities outside school hours) and different time periods (e.g. fall, spring). The results of analysis of the information from both formal and informal assessments provide the basis for outlining a program to teach social skills and promote social integration.

There is one caution which must be recognized as the collaborative team collects assessment data. As professionals bring their collective views to focus on one child there may be a tendency to over identify areas of concern or need relevant to the child's social and cognitive development. This may have an overwhelming and discouraging effect upon some members of the team, particularly parents and the classroom teachers who work with the student everyday. Early in the planning stage, the collaborative team needs to identify the student's areas of strength and set priorities for programming. Social skill needs which could be associated with social immaturity or a lack of opportunity to practice and refine specific behaviours may be recorded for future consideration but not specifically addressed as an immediate programming need. A strength of the collaborative team is its potential to enhance a consistent instructional approach to identified needs and to outline long-term programming needs.

Social Skills Training

The instruction of a number of compensatory skills (e.g. braille, orientation and mobility, daily living skills) have traditionally been associated with appropriate educational programming for those with a visual impairment. Given the findings of research and the reports of educators and parents relevant to the social competence and acceptance of children with a visual impairment, it is imperative that the instruction of social skills be considered a compulsory area of instruction for these students. Furthermore, it must be assumed that the majority of children with a visual impairment will need routine, formal intervention throughout their school years to ensure their social/emotional development needs are addressed. Examples of social skills which may be specifically required by children with a visual impairment are the ability to

- explain visual impairment to others using age-appropriate vocabulary
- outline implications visual impairment has for performance of daily routines and activities both in and outside school environment
- generate potential solutions to problems of access to visual information and to participation in typical activities of peers

- be aware of mannerisms, know how they are perceived by others, and control them in the presence of others
- be aware of and maintain appropriate posture (e.g., sitting in class)
- make eye contact and/or direct gaze toward listener
- understand the concept of nonverbal communication and its importance to those who are fully sighted
- maintain appropriate distance between self and person with whom interacting
- initiate actions which provide cues to appropriate responses which help to put individuals who are sighted at ease (e.g., reaches out to shake hands)
- be aware of and seek opportunities to help others
- use appropriate speech rhythms (e.g., response latency, the length of time from end of a prompt to the beginning of the response).

The following suggestions should be taken into consideration when planning the implementation of a social skills training program:

1. All children in the classroom will benefit from social skills training. As much as possible, social skills training for students with a visual impairment should be incorporated within group instruction provided to all children in the classroom.
2. As children grow and develop so does the complexity and variety of social skills they require to interact effectively in their social environments. Students with a visual impairment need routine and on-going instruction and monitoring of their social skills to ensure their changing needs are being addressed. Inclusion of social skill goals in the student's individualized education program helps to ensure parents and educators are monitoring and evaluating social development in the same manner as academic progress.
3. The student with a visual impairment should be involved in the planning of social skills training and the strategies used to practice and refine these skills. The integrity of the student must be protected by being sensitive to individual differences, respecting one's right to privacy, accommodating cultural practices of those from different backgrounds, and providing feedback and information in a candid but diplomatic manner.
4. When teaching social skills, incorporate a variety of instructional methods such as discussion, coaching, task analysis, self-monitoring, behaviourial contracts, peer-mediation, modelling, and role playing. Students with a visual impairment may sometimes require hand-over-hand assistance to develop a kinaesthetic awareness of a particular skill (e.g., extending one's hand to initiate a handshake).
5. To realize long-term changes in the social skills of students with a visual impairment, those aspects of the social environment which enhance and detract from the social acceptance of these students must be identified and

altered to provide a receptive learning environment in which to practice and refine newly acquired skills.

6. Ensure parents are aware of the specific social skills which are being practised in school so they may encourage the student's use of these skills during interaction in the home and in the community.

Choosing an appropriate social skills training program can be an onerous task given the abundance of resource material presently available. One highly recommended program written specifically for children and youth with a visual impairment is entitled *Independent Living: A Curriculum with Adaptations for Students with Visual Impairments* by R. Loumiet and N. Levack. The first volume, entitled *Social Competence*, outlines program goals in instructional areas such as social interaction, self-concept, nonverbal communication, personal/social sexuality, and scholastic success. Volume II, *Self-Care and Maintenance of Personal Environment,* addresses areas such as dressing, hygiene, eating, housekeeping, health and safety, and self-advocacy. Finally, Volume III, *Play and Leisure*, deals with topics such as management of leisure time, social play, physical games and sports, and science and technology. This curriculum is both a resource and a guide for assessment, programming, and instruction in the area of independent living and social development. Each area has stated goals with the related skills outlined in appropriate age levels. Checklists for each area are provided along with lesson plans and a wealth of information about adapted materials, special teaching methods, instructional materials and resources for teaching ideas and activities. *The Independent Living Curriculum*, in conjunction with the book entitled *The Development of Social Skills by Blind and Visually Impaired Students* by S. Sacks, L. Kekelis, and R. Gaylord-Ross, provides a comprehensive resource for use in planning social skills programs for students with a visual impairment.

Social skills programs written for students at specific age levels (e.g., *Skillstreaming the Adolescent* by Goldstein, Sprafkin, Gershaw, and Klein) may also be suitable resources upon which to base overall programming. Also, programs that address impairments other than those visual in nature may offer some useful information (e.g., *Making Better Choices: A Curriculum for Teaching Cognitive Planning and Social Skills to Improve Social and Academic Behavior* by Harris). An extensive list of social skills training programs is provided in Appendix B.

Understanding Visual Impairment

Children with a visual impairment need to be knowledgable about their visual impairment. They should have an age appropriate understanding of the basic anatomy and physiology of the eye, the name of the eye condition, and factors which affect their visual efficiency (e.g., lighting, contrast, print size). It is essential that they be able to provide a reasonable explanation of their eye condition and its implications to others. Periodic elaboration of the conceptual and practical aspects of their visual impairment will be required as they mature. Early in the adolescent years, counselling to address any genetic considerations associated with a student's eye condition should be provided. It is only through awareness and education that these students can learn to accept their impairment and demonstrate a sense of self-acceptance to others.

From an early age children with a visual impairment should be encouraged to search for solutions to problems of visual access or ways to complete activities which require some adaptations to accommodate their visual impairment. Children who display self-initiative and self-advocacy are less likely to become victims of learned helplessness. If they develop a problem-solving approach to accessing information, their teachers and peers will also feel more comfortable and capable of accommodating someone with a visual impairment. Practice in generating solutions to accommodate their visual impairment will help children develop a belief that they can do most activities and decrease the likelihood that they routinely avoid activities they feel may be too difficult or impossible for one with a visual impairment. Teachers with special training in the education of those with a visual impairment are often good role models or sources of information in this area.

Visual Impairment as a Label of Primary Potency

Those who have had the opportunity to work with a group of children who are visually impaired will have noticed how insignificant visual impairment becomes when all participants are visually impaired. In such situations, the focus of conversation is upon the activity at hand or common interests such as sports, music, or video games. In an integrated setting where there is usually only one person with a visual impairment, this aspect of the individual generally becomes a primary focus of attention and concern. Children with visual impairments may learn to think of themselves primarily in terms of their impairment while other aspects of their being (e.g., interest in science, skill in gymnastics, pleasant personality) seem insignificant by comparison. One of the greatest challenges facing educators and parents of children with a visual impairment is that of orchestrating an environment in which visual impairment can be candidly and openly discussed without it becoming the most prominent attribute of these students. The following suggestions provide some guidance in reaching this goal:

1. Take every opportunity to discuss similarities students with a visual impairment share with their peers. For example, in the presence of peers initiate conversations about the interests of the student who is visually impaired, what was watched on television, or what activities the family enjoyed on an outing. This will provide the student's peers accurate information about the similarities between themselves and the student with a visual impairment.
2. When arranging for class outings, guest speakers, or substitute teachers, inform people of the student's visual impairment and how to respond to or accommodate it prior to the activity. This will decrease the likelihood

that the visual impairment will become a stress-producing or negative aspect of the activity. As well, overt discussion of appropriate ways to accommodate the student with a visual impairment will model the expectation that this individual is to be meaningfully involved and a contributing member of the class.

3. Discourage the development of a special status associated with being visually impaired. Invariably, "the novelty wears off" and students with a visual impairment who have been given special recognition or attention because of their visual impairment find themselves isolated in the mainstream. Accomplishments and successes of students with a visual impairment should be acknowledged in the same way as those of their peers. Adults should take care not to exaggerate the accomplishments of these children or to lower standards to ensure success. Actions as simple as the principal always speaking to the student with a visual impairment and not to classmates contributes to the creation of a special status which inevitably detracts from the student's social acceptance. Remember, the importance of peer acceptance to children increases significantly as they proceed through elementary school. Unwarranted adult attention can detract from acceptance by classmates.
4. Redirect conversation to other topics if students routinely initiate discussion of their visual impairment. Unfortunately for some students, their visual impairment becomes the focus of their lives. It may be necessary to have a candid discussion with the student about the need to develop and discuss interests which can be shared with peers.
5. Make adaptations required to provide access to learning materials prior to the presentation of the lesson. During a lesson when models are readily available or large print copies of handouts are distributed in conjunction with the distribution of materials to other students, inclusion of students with a visual impairment is demonstrated to be natural and spontaneous. Activities which are difficult to adapt or are inappropriate for students with a visual impairment need not be avoided. However, alternate activities incorporating similar or adapted learning objectives should be provided. Such an approach allows classmates a choice of activities and the student with a visual impairment the opportunity to participate in a meaningful activity associated with the topic of the lesson.
6. When appropriate, adults should verbalize their mistakes or personal weaknesses which pose difficulties for them. Such statements as "my writing was so messy I couldn't read it" or "I usually have difficulty finding my car in mall parking lots" help students with a visual impairment realize that all people have strengths and weaknesses which they must deal with on a daily basis. Frequently children with a visual impairment will blame all their problems (e.g., not having a friend, being a poor reader, not winning the race) on the impairment and avoid addressing aspects of their personality or behaviour which could improve their performance.

Caution must be taken not to discourage the open discussion of visual impairment which increases awareness and reduces the stigma frequently associated with blindness. The intent is to increase the awareness of both students with a visual impairment and their peers that there are more similarities between them than differences and that a visual impairment must not preclude the opportunity to "really get to know" the person with a visual impairment.

Preventing Learned Helplessness

When a student with a visual impairment is first enroled in an integrated setting, teachers usually voice concerns associated with such things as the child's safety, their ability to meet the special learning needs of the student, and the availability of time to prepare adapted materials or lessons. Responses to these concerns generally involve the use of peers to help the student with a visual impairment and/or the assignment of a teacher assistant to help both the teacher and the student. While neither of these responses is faulty in its original intent, what happens too frequently is that the amount of assistance offered the student does not change in response to the increasing competence of the student. A primary level student, initially requiring a guide to travel to the washroom, will not need to be escorted after having mastered the mobility skills to travel independently. Similarly, because of inappropriate expectations and/or pressures to meet the many time constraints of the school day, students with a visual impairment may be given too much unnecessary assistance with tasks they are capable of completing independently. A senior elementary student with a visual impairment may have a peer packing and unpacking her/his school bag in order to meet routine school timelines (e.g., catching the bus at 2:45 p.m.).

There are several negative consequences resulting from the provision of unwarranted help to students with a visual impairment. The primary one is that they learn to rely on assistance and do not practice the essential skills required to become independent. It is important to note that classmates frequently grow tired of volunteering or being assigned to help and begin to resent this obligation. Additionally, students with a visual impairment may associate the impairment with dependence upon others (e.g., a teacher/student aide) and develop the belief that they have limited control over their lives. Even as preschoolers, children with a visual impairment need to be given responsibilities which demonstrate their competence and the expectation that they are capable of taking control of their learning. They should be encouraged to take the responsibility to initiate contact with peers, seek out playmates, and gracefully refuse assistance which is not required. Of utmost importance, adults must facilitate opportunities for students with a visual impairment to help others. Both in the classroom and the community, these students need to experience the pleasure of helping others. This not only sends a powerful message to peers and the public in general, but has tremendous positive effects upon the self-esteem of the student.

Affiliation with Adults

A child becomes a member of a group when enroled in school and assigned to a given classroom. Because significant amounts of time are spent working and playing with the same children, the child develops a sense of belonging to this group, that is, a social identity based on participation with classmates. It is only through routine, positive interaction with members of the class that a student develops this sense of belonging and allegiance to the classroom group.

Many children with a visual impairment encounter difficulties in estab-lishing a social identity with a peer group. During the preschool years they are more likely than children who are fully sighted to spend significant amounts of time with adults, as most early intervention programs usually involve one-to-one instruction by an adult (e.g., teacher, therapist). When they are enroled in a preschool program outside the home, an adult assistant is frequently assigned to work with the student or the group has a low teacher-student ratio — again increasing the likelihood of contact with adults rather than peers. After they begin their formal education, there is additional adult contact provided to the student with a visual impairment by the teacher for the visually impaired, the orientation and mobility instructor, and, in many cases, a classroom teacher assistant. Because learning through imitation is often difficult for children with a severe visual impairment, routine adult intervention to provide instruction is a typical approach for these students.

A second consideration which may be seen to contribute to the tendency of students with a visual impairment to interact more frequently with adults is the tendency for them to experience developmental delays in both physical agility and social competence. Therefore, the child may have difficulty participating in the rough-and-tumble games of the elementary school playground with their peers, as well as lack the social skills which contribute to positive interaction with classmates during school activities. In both situations, the intervention to overcome these difficulties tends to be one-to-one instruction by an adult. Over a period of time, the student may become most comfortable when interacting with adults because they seldom respond in a negative way, are usually approachable, friendly and effective listeners, and do not run away. This tendency for students with a visual impairment to relate more effectively to adults than to peers emphasizes the importance of involving classmates of these students in programs to teach them social skills and to increase their social interaction.

Organization Skills

As students with a visual impairment have moved from small, segregated classes for the visually impaired to integrated placements where classroom enrolments are much larger, there is an increased need for them to develop organization skills required in an integrated setting and to perform with a comparable level of teacher-student interaction provided other students. A frequent complaint of classroom teachers who have a student with a visual impairment is the tendency this student has to slow the pace of classroom activities. Based on observation of integrated settings, it is apparent that these students can increase their efficiency through practice and mastery of such basic organization skills as the following:

- using bookmarks to locate place in timely manner
- storing loose papers in an indexed three ring binder
- organizing book shelves with most frequently used texts in one area
- labelling all books and binders so they can be distinguished quickly
- using various methods to label materials for future identification
- keeping work area uncluttered and organized so as to have quick access to books and materials
- getting materials necessary for next lesson without prompting
- working quickly and accurately
- using techniques to maximize visual efficiency
- self-initiating use of aids/materials which enhance efficiency
- reading directions before beginning task
- asking questions to clarify assignment before beginning it
- keeping copies of schedules in school bag and in desk
- bringing needed materials to class
- putting paper in braille writer/typewriter/printer in timely manner
- refraining from mannerisms which decrease working rate
- independently packing and unpacking book bag
- using self-initiative in obtaining access to visual information
- working independently for extended periods of time
- requesting assistance only after attempting to solve problem independently
- travelling independently and with ease throughout the classroom
- putting on and removing outside clothing and footwear in a timely manner
- using available adaptations, e.g., shoes with velcro straps if unable to independently tie sneakers.

It should be noted that many of these skills are those which would be encouraged in all students. However, students with a visual impairment frequently are not expected to master these organizational skills or many of them are done for them. Mastery and efficient performance of organization skills should have a high priority when establishing individualized education plans for these students.

Nonverbal Communication

Under the discussion of social skills, the importance of learning to incorporate aspects of nonverbal communication, such as gestures or facial expressions, was discussed. However, classmates and those who work with students with a visual impairment must develop an appreciation for the aspects of nonverbal communication which are problematic for one with a severe visual impairment and the effect this may have on the way this individual interacts with others. If classmates know that the student with a visual impairment does not see a friendly wave or must direct her/his gaze to the right of the speaker to see facial expressions, hopefully they will not interpret the student's behaviour in a negative way. Informed adults and classmates can learn to spontaneously provide students with a visual impairment with access to nonverbal information by verbalizing events as they take place or by precuing the student to attend to a specific situation.

Of equal importance is the need for adults and classmates to provide these students with verbal feedback relevant to both behaviours which others consider to be appropriate and inappropriate. Because students with a visual impairment have limited access to visual information they may not be able to imitate body postures which are considered acceptable or which invite interaction with others. Formal instruction or purposeful comments can provide the student with knowledge which others gain through incidental learning. As well, the response to mannerisms which are perceived by others to be atypical or "weird" behaviours should be candidly discussed with students with a visual impairment.

Another aspect of nonverbal communication to be considered when working with students who are visually impaired is the existence of some communication patterns which require quick and accurate responses to visual information and which will be, for the most part, difficult for those with a visual impairment to accommodate. Students with a visual impairment, for example, have difficulty scanning the cafeteria to locate the group of friends with whom they wish to sit. Similarly, when participating in group discussions, the timing of conversation in conjunction with nonverbal messages, such as nodding the head or directing the gaze toward the person who is intended to speak next, are messages that will not be received, hence accurately responded to by one with a visual impairment. The awkwardness which sometimes results is inevitable and may be an appropriate topic for discussion with older students. What is important is that the classmates of students with a visual impairment learn to accept such situations as the consequence of missed visual information rather than interpreting this as inappropriate behaviour or disinterest in interaction on the part of the student who is visually impaired.

Access to Information

One of the most pervasive consequences of having a visual impairment is the potential limitation it places on access to information, particularly that essential to spontaneous learning through observation and imitation. The majority of information received is through the visual sense. Therefore, one of the greatest challenges for educators and parents of children with a visual impairment is to provide access to information. This enormous task is further complicated by the need to determine the gaps in a child's current learning which interfere with new learning. Accessing knowledge which is not readily available (e.g., behaviour patterns which are valued by a given age group), is also an issue requiring careful consideration and creative solutions. Examples of the types of information which students with a visual impairment may require assistance in accessing are

- unwritten rules of pupil culture, such as those things to tell teachers and those things which are shared only by children
- activities which are popular on the playground and the rules which guide participation
- the opportunities which exist for interaction with peers outside the classroom, such as debating club, choral groups, school newspaper, and recreational pursuits
- the types of problems other students are experiencing as they proceed through school (e.g., peer pressure, belonging, understanding others)
- common knowledge items such as the current fashions in clothing, hairstyles, television programs, music, and recreational and leisure pursuits
- popular games (e.g., board games, card games, video games) and how to play them
- how to participate and what to do on playground equipment, how to participate in run and chase games, how to play in a group
- information which is displayed on classroom walls, bulletin boards, overhead projectors, film screens, and television monitors.

There is a definite correlation between the frequency of interaction with peers and the likelihood that students with a visual impairment will be exposed to the types of information listed above. It is during routine interaction with peers that many of these topics are discussed. Thus, the student who is isolated from routine positive interaction with peers will be at risk both socially and academically.

Self-Esteem

Integrated settings which do not plan for and monitor the social acceptance of students with a visual impairment create a potentially hostile social environment for these children. Perhaps the most significant implication for students with a visual impairment is the risk to the development of a positive self-esteem. We cannot "give" someone high self-esteem because it is a consequence of the myriad of practices and experience which promote acceptance, understanding, caring, and respect. It is not that the conditions or techniques to promote high self-esteem are different for students with a visual impairment than for their classmates. However, when social integration is left to chance, frequently students do not experience a positive acceptance of difference, may be misunderstood and/or misinterpret messages from others, feel isolated or rejected by peers, and may encounter lowered expectations and false praise. It is too often assumed that social acceptance will happen spontaneously or does not need to be explicitly addressed.

Consider the subtle messages received by students with a visual impairment when they are usually the last ones chosen for a partner, when they are not given a copy of the class handout, when they routinely spend their recess alone on the swing, when they do not see the teacher's smile or nod of approval, when adults are unable to provide information about the types of careers available to them, when parents become exasperated with the extra time and effort required to attend to their visual needs, and when people often ask what is "wrong" with their eyesight. None of these outcomes are intended but are inevitable without careful monitoring of the type and frequency of negative messages associated with visual impairment received by these students who are attempting to conform to an environment developed for and by those who are fully sighted. In addition to the usual strategies for facilitating the development of positive self-esteem in all children, the following suggestions will provide information necessary to address the unique needs of those with a visual impairment:

1. Monitor the frequency and type of peer interaction experienced by students with a visual impairment to determine the nature of this interaction.
2. Locate successful role models with a visual impairment who can act as a source of encouragement for students with a visual impairment and their parents.
3. During White Cane Week have a school display of famous people with a visual impairment and their contributions throughout history. Demonstrate technology which promotes independence and/or invite guest speakers with a visual impairment.
4. Arrange for students to spend time with others who are visually impaired (e.g., weekend camps, friendship groups) so they may share and learn from the experiences of one another.
5. Provide assertiveness training and opportunities for self-advocacy when the student is young.
6. When appropriate, have students participate in developing their individualized education plans and become involved in case conferences or other relevant meetings.
7. Ensure playgrounds and classrooms have available recreational and learning activities which provide the opportunity for students with a visual impairment to participate actively and competently.

8. Ensure expectations for student performance, both social and academic, are appropriate.
9. Involve the student in setting goals, thereby providing opportunities for the student to experience a sense of achievement and independence in reaching these goals.
10. Invite parents to participate in learning opportunities which focus on enhancing self-esteem because parents play a primary role in nurturing self-esteem in their children.

To ensure the opportunity for students with a visual impairment to develop high self-esteem, it is critical to provide a context which emphasizes the abilities and minimizes the limitations imposed by visual impairment.

For further information on the enhancement of self-esteem and available assessment and programming materials, a list of references is provided in Appendix C.

Praise and Encouragement

The negative aspects of false praise for students with a visual impairment were mentioned earlier in this chapter. Receiving praise for performance that is not worthy or credible can lead to confusion about what is acceptable or even possible in relation to one's performance. However, praise in general is known to have some detrimental effects upon the behaviour of children. Routine teacher praise as an external reward may interfere, for example, with the child's development of intrinsic or internal motivation such as self-satisfaction in a job well done. The externally motivated child who depends upon praise from others requires immediate gratification and may cease working when this is not forthcoming. In the group or classroom situation, praise may stimulate rivalry and competition as opposed to cooperation. The student who is fortunate enough to receive the teacher's praise has a sense of superiority while those who have not yet been praised may feel unjustly treated. Adults, in their enthusiasm to be helpful and supportive of children with a visual impairment, may use praise when encouragement would be far more beneficial to the child. Encouragement can be given during the task, when the task is completed, or even if the child has made a conscientious effort but failed (e.g., I'm sure you can solve this problem, now where do you think the trouble is?). When the child accomplishes something which may be trivial for other children (e.g., independently travelling to the washroom and back) encouragement such as "you must be pleased with yourself" is obviously more appropriate than praise such as "you are terrific". The use of encouragement helps to build a trusting relationship in which the student is not afraid to try or to risk failure. Evaluation of the child is not inherent with the use of encouragement, hence, there is a sense of being accepted as one is. This, in itself, is a tremendous boost to one's self-esteem. The following phrases are examples of encouraging comments:

- I'm sure you can solve this problem but if you need help...
- You do a good job of....
- You must be pleased with your work.
- We like you but we don't like it when you....
- So you made a mistake; what can you learn from that mistake?
- You did very well on the exam.
- You work with such enthusiasm. Any teacher would enjoy having you in class.

When examining important aspects relevant to the social integration of students with a visual impairment, it is evident that many are related and often interdependent. For example, developing good organization skills assists the student to demonstrate competence and independence, experiences which simultaneously enhance positive self-esteem. Students are more likely to receive positive feedback and even encouragement when they are actively involved with others as opposed to sitting alone. Encouragement plays a significant role in promoting a willingness to try in students with a visual impairment.

The routine use of encouragement rather than praise may be initially difficult to incorporate within one's spontaneous responses. The use of praise is usually more familiar to educators and parents. Therefore, it is helpful if adults attempt to self-monitor their use of encouragement with students with a visual impairment as well as requesting relevant feedback from other adults in the school or home.

To assist in outlining the considerations relevant to students with a visual impairment, a checklist is provided in Appendix D.

Considerations Relevant to Classmates of Students with a Visual Impairment

When adults discuss the interaction of children and youth it is not uncommon to hear someone say "children can be cruel" in reference to the seemingly insensitive comments which children may make to one another. Yet, it is only through the process of interaction that children experiment with, practice and refine social interaction skills. Making cruel comments or displaying aggressive behaviours are steps in the learning process leading to more acceptable social responses. Through exposure and practice children learn to refrain from making comments which will offend others and develop nonaggressive responses in reaction to the undesirable behaviour of others. Social cognition, like cognitive development, is a dynamic process which varies from individual to individual and reflects the influences of numerous variables in a child's environment (e.g., home situation, learning structures in the school) as well as those specific to a given child (e.g., temperament). In attempting to enhance the social acceptance of students with a visual impairment, the role played by their peers is an influential one. Recommended programming for the classmates of students with a visual impairment is presented in the following section.

Knowledge of Visual Impairment

Children are naturally curious about new or unfamiliar aspects of their environment. In schools where a student with a visual impairment has been integrated, it is not uncommon to see children experimenting to determine the visual abilities or other skills of their classmate who is visually impaired. Holding up fingers for the student who is visually impaired to count or moving objects in proximity of this person to observe if there is a visual response are typical of this type of behaviour. Most times these actions are not intended to be unkind or stressful for the student with a visual impairment, even though viewed by adults as being such, rather they are prompted by a desire to know about the impairment.

A knowledge of visual impairment and its implications are essential if the classmates of students with a visual impairment are to develop accurate perceptions of these students. They should be aware of the nature of a given student's impairment, implications of this impairment both in the classroom and on the playground, and the differing implications of the various types of visual impairment. If classmates are to accurately interpret the behaviour of students with a visual impairment they must have insight into how this student perceives the environment. For example, when classmates know a playmate can not observe what is happening in a group, they can spontaneously provide information which will encourage or enable the student with a visual impairment to participate. Classmates can be taught to substitute nonverbal communication, such as a wave of the hand, with verbal greetings. As well, classmates can be a very valuable part of the problem-solving team in matters directly associated with peer interaction and how best to include students with a visual impairment in activities outside the classroom. They know the rules of pupil culture and will most often generate solutions which do not infringe upon the perceived rights of others. As has been mentioned previously, with knowledge comes understanding.

Open Discussion of Visual Impairment

As adults we can rationalize our thinking about visual impairment and seek information about its etiology or other questions which arise. Children do not have the same avenues open to satisfy their curiosity. They are dependent upon adults not only for access to much of this information but also to legitimize those topics which are suitable for exploration or discussion. When visual impairment is not a topic for open, spontaneous, and natural discussion in the home and in the classroom, children, both classmates and students with a visual impairment, interpret this awkwardness as an indication that visual impairment is bad, immoral, or something for which one should feel ashamed. Understandably, classmates cannot appreciate either the differences or similarities of peers with a visual impairment if they do not understand the impairment and its social implications and do not have the freedom to openly discuss questions or concerns as they arise.

Strategies for Involving Classmates in Promoting Social Integration

In schools where affective education and cooperative learning are prominent aspects of the learning environment, considerable emphasis will have been placed on the positive acceptance of difference and social acceptance of all children. Exposure to adults who model appropriate respect for and interaction with students who are visually impaired is, of course, a prerequisite for social integration. Since social integration is primarily integration into the world of one's peers, classmates must become an informed and integral part of the integration process. Programs to enhance social integration will, therefore, benefit from the formal involvement of peers. Some of the ways peers may be involved are in peer-mediated social skills training, peer mentoring, and peer support groups.

Teaching social skills to students with a visual impairment through peer-mediation involves the training of peers as social skills instructors (Sacks, Kekelis & Gaylord-Ross, 1992). They receive information about the child's visual impairment and its potential influence on behaviour, as well as on how to model appropriate social responses in their interactions with this child. Although the specific arrangements may vary, the peer instructor is usually prepared to address one or two specific social behaviours during a scheduled meeting time with the student. During the meeting time the peer instructor participates in an activity with the student with a visual impairment and during this interaction provides direct instruction, encouragement, and modelling of appropriate behaviour. For example, a peer instructor assisting the student with a visual impairment to direct her gaze toward the speaker, might say, "How about turning your head toward me when you talk to me." Peer-mediated instruction usually results in greater generalization of the newly acquired skills to situations outside the instructional period than does similar instruction by the teacher.

Peer mentoring is most often a strategy used at the junior and senior high levels. It involves the assignment of a student with advanced skills in a given area to a student who requires assistance in this area or needs encouragement to realize their potential in this area. For students with a visual impairment, this might entail having a classmate recruit, encourage, and nurture the participation of this student in an extracurricular activity such as the debating club, choir, or band. The focus of the peer mentoring could also be on improving social acceptance, increasing the frequency of social interaction, or modeling appropriate social behaviour. The student acting as the mentor receives training in the mentoring process as well as assistance in addressing specific difficulties which might be interfering with the successful participation of the student with a visual impairment. Often the student mentor becomes a strong advocate for the student who is visually impaired as well as a role model for other students in the school. It is critical that educators remember to identify the skills possessed by the student who is visually impaired so that he/she can be assigned to assist other students in the school.

There are a variety of peer support programs which can provide invaluable assistance to students with a visual impairment. In large schools where there are several students with similar disabilities, a support group to address social integration issues may be viable. In most schools, peer support groups provide scheduled times when students meet to openly discuss any variety of personal concerns such as social acceptance, school or family problems, or academic difficulties. Groups may be organized and lead by either a teacher or a student leader. Student leaders have training in effective listening, problem-solving strategies, and identification of problems requiring professional assistance. Groups establish rules with which participants must comply, such as keeping all discussions of the group confidential, not making value judgements, and not allowing putdowns. Students with a visual impairment who participate in such groups have first-hand exposure to the types of problems common to many teenagers, fully sighted or visually impaired.

The formal involvement of peers in promoting social integration provides invaluable experiences for both students with a visual impairment and their classmates. The peers have an opportunity to broaden their understanding of visual impairment and to develop a meaningful relationship with this student. Students with a visual impairment have first-hand access to the rules and practices of the pupil culture in which they are immersed and have an opportunity to interact with their peers in a more risk-free setting than is usually available. In all programs involving peer assistance, care must be taken to ensure the ongoing respect for the integrity of the student with a visual impairment. This student must not become "the class project" but must be included by virtue of a belief in the positive acceptance of difference and in the value of all children.

To assist in the outlining of the considerations relevant to classmates of students with a visual impairment, a checklist is provided in Appendix D.

Additional Suggestions for Parents and Teachers

Many of the suggestions for teachers and parents, although directed specifically toward the integration of children who are visually impaired, have the potential to enhance the affective development of all children. Many are applicable to either the home or the school situation. In using lists of suggestions such as the following, it is important to remember that one's understanding of a given student will act as a guide in the implementation of those suggestions which are appropriate for this student in given situations. Hopefully, the needs of individual students at various times in their school careers and social development will dictate the most appropriate types of intervention.

Suggestions for Classroom Teachers

1. Seek opportunities to explore personal feelings and beliefs about those with a visual impairment prior to enroling a student with a visual impairment in your class. Acknowledging some of the negative aspects associated with blindness better enables identification and adoption of attitudinal changes required to model the positive acceptance of difference for all students.
2. Encourage the principal or designated administrator to take responsibility for providing the school level leadership required to enhance the social acceptance and instructional progress of students with a visual impairment.
3. Substitute teachers who will be taking over classes when teachers are absent should be familiar with the student with a visual impairment and her/his learning needs. Where possible, substitute teachers should participate in case conferences and professional development activities which are designed to address this student's needs and to promote the social integration of students with disabilities.
4. Plan to include students with a visual impairment in all activities. To enhance their participation provide enough structure so they can anticipate what is going to happen next. Materials requiring brailling, enlarging or other formatting should be available for distribution when other students receive their copies. When the planned activity is not suitable for the student with a visual impairment, alternate activities with similar objectives should be planned in advance and accessible when needed. Do not be afraid to acknowledge that a particular activity is inappropriate for an individual with a visual impairment but describe it as "inappropriate" rather than something this student "cannot do".
5. Organize the classroom and the storage of equipment and material to enhance the mobility, independence, and efficiency of the student with a visual impairment.
6. Make use of the many resources available from the teacher of the visually impaired. Have this specialist preview your lesson plans and textbooks and routinely observe in your classroom to make suggestions for enhancing the affective and cognitive development of the student with a visual impairment. Inquire about ways to incorporate the special instruction in such areas as orientation and mobility or computer technology in your classroom to assist the student in meaningful practice of new skills.
7. Encourage the teacher for the visually impaired to provide instruction in the regular classroom whenever possible. Inform classmates of the types of activities in which their classmate with a visual impairment is involved when instruction is provided outside the classroom. Accurate information relevant to the special instructional needs of the student with a visual impairment increases the knowledge and understanding of classmates.
8. Prior to the actual assignment of a teacher or student assistant in your classroom, consider the most effective use of this staff member and the

potential interference with social integration created when an assistant is expected to be with one child throughout most of the day. Meet with the classroom assistant and establish roles and responsibilities prior to introduction to the classroom. Work together to promote the social and academic development of the student with a visual impairment.

9. During the first week of school provide a variety of activities to increase a sense of familiarity among the students. Provide the student with a visual impairment with a list of the names of classmates. Younger students should receive a tape recording of the voices of each classmate to assist in early identification of classmates. Develop the habit of calling on students by name rather than gestures such as pointing.
10. Alternate group seating arrangements and group membership for various activities to ensure all students have an opportunity to become well acquainted with the student with a visual impairment and this student with all classmates.
11. Provide a variety of games and learning activities which entice other children to participate with the student with a visual impairment. Consider the type of interaction encouraged by different activities. For example, individual activities such as colouring involves less interaction than imaginary play or activities requiring cooperation.
12. When preparing lesson plans consider the program adaptations which are the least isolating for students with a visual impairment. Analyze the dilemmas associated with developing independence and the use of special equipment or techniques. Flexible guidelines which accommodate such dilemmas need to be established. For example, having a student travel with a sighted guide to the cafeteria increases the probability that the student will eat with classmates. Opportunities for independent travel can be easily found during other parts of the school day.
13. The social issues encountered by students vary from one age group to another. Ensure strategies to enhance social acceptance and solutions to difficulties with interaction are age appropriate. For example, teenagers might need some assistance in finding transportation alternatives because they cannot drive a car. A younger student might be interested in investigating adaptations which would enhance participation in a particular sport.
14. Encourage students with a visual impairment to participate in activities which increase their exposure to peers (e.g., participation in extra-curricular activities, working in the cafeteria or on the school newspaper).
15. Provide opportunities for students with a visual impairment to choose a partner for work or leisure activities. However, as a matter of practice, preassign students to groups or partnerships to limit the likelihood of the same children being routinely chosen last.
16. Identify those classmates who are receptive to working and playing with students with a visual impairment and those classmates who appeal to these students. Orchestrate opportunities for these mutually accepting par-

ties to work and play together. Refrain from assigning the same students to routinely interact with the student with a visual impairment.

17. Promote the maintenance of class friendship groups when student placements are being considered for the upcoming school year. Students who appear to be isolated from the group should be placed with peers who appear to be most receptive to this student.

Suggestions for Teachers of the Visually Impaired

1. Make observation of the interaction of the student a priority. The knowledge and experience which the teacher of the visually impaired brings from experience with a number of students with a visual impairment is an invaluable source of both insight and potential solutions to social integration difficulties. It is also essential to monitor the degree of access to information and meaningful learning being experienced by the student in the integrated setting. While observing, take note of needed adaptations or strategies which would enhance the participation of the student in classroom and playground activities.
2. Provide simulators (i.e., goggles with lenses that simulate various eye conditions such as reduced acuity, cataracts, or restrictions of peripheral vision) which represent the visual condition of the student. These may be used for instructional periods with both adults and classmates. Simulators provide firsthand exposure to visual impairment and its implications in the student's environment, thus assist others to generate solutions to problems which may arise.
3. Nurture a positive working relationship with the student's classroom teachers. A relationship which is characterized by mutual respect, trust, sharing, and cooperative efforts on behalf of the student will have significant benefits for the student.
4. Allow classmates to use the special equipment and materials provided for the student with a visual impairment. This exposure will increase awareness of the adaptations used by this student as well as help to eliminate the special status associated with them.
5. Provide instruction to the student in the regular classroom whenever possible. Include classmates in learning activities, even those which are devoted to special compensatory skills required by those with a visual impairment (e.g. learning braille, operating a CCTV). Such activities provide demonstrations of the competent performance of the student with a visual impairment and increase the awareness and understanding of classmates.
6. Assist classroom teachers in the open discussion of visual impairment and its implications. It takes time and exposure for adults to become comfortable with this process.
7. Develop a collection of games and learning activities (e.g. braille edition of scrabble or monopoly, electronic question and answer games with

speech output) which promote the social and instructional inclusion of students with a visual impairment. Make these available to classroom teachers.

8. Identify activities which will entice classmates of the student with a visual impairment to initiate interaction or to join the student in an activity.
9. In conjunction with parents of the student with a visual impairment, discuss and practice how the student can communicate visual needs to others in a polite, forthright manner. Encourage the adoption of language and terms which will clarify such explanations.
10. Be alert for signs of frustration or concern being experienced by classroom teachers. Allow them an opportunity to verbalize their concerns and assist them in generating possible solutions to problems which arise.
11. Actively pursue class placements for students with a visual impairment which address affective education, promote the development of high self-esteem, and incorporate cooperative learning structures.
12. Acknowledge the expertise parents and educators have in their given areas (e.g. physical education, language arts, parenting) and request their feedback relevant to the appropriateness of recommendations made to accommodate the student's needs in a given subject or circumstance.
13. Emphasize the importance of spending instructional time with the student to teach social skills required to participate competently in both in-class and extra-curricular activities (e.g. playground games, board games, school newspaper).
14. Become familiar with the most popular activities and interests in the student's particular classroom. Use this information to introduce the student to these activities or to inspire interest in similar pursuits.
15. Practice age appropriate conversational skills with the student. Identify appropriate topics for discussion with peers and introduce new interests which are emerging within the classroom so the student will have the necessary information and skills to interact successfully.
16. Seek out teaching strategies, methods, and activities which enhance the active participation of students with a visual impairment in an integrated setting. Share these with both teachers and parents.
17. Provide teachers with models and other adapted materials which both assist the student with a visual impairment and make the lesson more interesting for classmates.
18. Provide classroom teachers with feedback relevant to the inclusion of the student with a visual impairment and the appropriateness of teaching methods and materials for this student. Make suggestions and acknowledge the teacher's incorporation of these.

Suggestions for Parents

1. Raising a child with a visual impairment requires much courage and perseverance. Use available resources to help provide both the physical and emotional support needed to become child advocates.

2. Insist on taking an active role in the planning and implementation of your child's program. Monitor both the academic progress and social acceptance and interaction. Ensure individualized education plans have appropriate goals in both areas.
3. Develop a support network or participate in a support group which can provide both moral support and generate potential solutions to difficulties as they arise. Each year in a child's development brings new issues and challenges. Make use of the expertise of other parents who have gone through the process with their children.
4. From an early age, encourage your child to become a self-advocate. Have her/him assume responsibilities at home, demonstrate assertive behaviour in the community, and gradually assume a primary role in dealing with eye specialists and agencies and organizations dealing with those with a visual impairment.
5. When your child is young, participate in parent-child programs where you can model the appropriate way to interact with a child with a visual impairment. As your child progresses to community activities for older children, be willing to assist leaders with initial planning to accommodate a child with a visual impairment.
6. Stay abreast of the language, music, television programs, dress, and fashions of the pupil culture in your child's school and neighbourhood. Observe during school and extra-curricular activities to become familiar with the interests of other children. Discuss these with your child and introduce toys, games, and other activities that are popular.
7. Plan activities which will encourage your child's interaction with classmates such as inviting them to play at your house or allowing her/him to take popular games to school.
8. Expose your child to the wealth of activities available in the community (e.g., youth groups, library sponsored activities, recreational pursuits, visits to fire hall, etc.). Encourage your child to become a volunteer or to assist in some aspect of community involvement.
9. Initiate discussions of relationship and friendships with your child (e.g., aspects of friendships). Encourage interest in others, complimenting the performance of others, and seeking their opinions. Role play conversations to practice such skills.
10. Use a checklist and set goals to master age appropriate daily living skills (e.g., dressing, eating, household chores). Help your child to develop organization strategies which enhance efficiency and time management.
11. Discourage mannerisms from an early age. Provide the child with candid feedback about how mannerisms are viewed by others. Use encouragement and positive feedback to help the child self-monitor her/his mannerisms and ensure teachers reinforce similar practices during school hours.
12. Limit the number of sedentary activities (e.g., watching television or listening to music) in which your child is involved. Use of the telephone, ham radio activities, and computer bulletin boards provide opportunities to in-

teract. Recreational pursuits which promote physical fitness are not only essential to good health but frequently provide opportunities for social interaction as well. When children are exposed to a variety of activities they develop a broad knowledge base, potential interests, and topics for conversations with peers.

Conclusion

If society is to make a sincere commitment to the integration of students with disabilities, great attention must be focused on the process of integration and on the complex philosophical, moral, and practical issues inherent in this concept. Educators and parents must identify the potential effects of integration upon the basic cultural assumptions present in schools and the incompatible aspects associated with the integration of these children. There are numerous circumstances and variables which interact to create unique situations in every classroom. Therefore, when considering actions to enhance the social acceptance and interaction of students with a visual impairment there can be no single solution or master program. What is required is a collaborative team comprised of administrators, educators, parents, and students. The main function of this team, that is, its mission, must be to enhance the social acceptance and interaction of students with a visual impairment. All members of the team must understand that the social/emotional development of these students may be a very different developmental experience from that of their peers, hence, may require new insights and approaches to social learning. All must realize that the affective development of these children must not be left to chance. Program planning and instruction to promote the social acceptance and interaction of students with a visual impairment has to be an essential component of their schooling experience.

8

Social Integration Issues in Our Schools

Introduction

Schools throughout North America are being confronted by a diversity of challenges never before encountered by the education system. Despite their efforts to meet a multiplicity of responsibilities, schools are routinely criticized for the failure of students in reaching acceptable levels of academic achievement and discipline. There is much talk of parent dissatisfaction with schools, the low morale of teachers, and the limited resources schools have available to meet the extraordinary expectations placed upon them. The problems facing schools are complex ones without easy solutions. Yet, in the midst of all the controversy there is usually a glimmer of hope — a school which has been able to tackle significant problems and regardless of great adversity achieve a remarkable degree of success. The philosophies these schools have propagated and the strategies they have implemented to achieve their goals serve as models for educators and parents who are willing to make the commitment to schools that welcome *all* students.

In this final chapter, four controversial issues associated with the social integration of students with a disability are presented. First, consideration will be given to the role of educators in facilitating the social skills development of their students. The second issue focuses upon the inclusion of children with multiple disabilities and a clarification of the expectations for their meaningful participation in our schools. Next, the significant role in enhancing social integration which can be played by paraprofessionals hired to assist students with a disability is considered. Finally, the need for adult intervention in structured playground activities to create an inclusive playground environment where the benefits of play are accessible to all children are presented. Hopefully, the information in this chapter will assist the reader to reflect upon new ways of viewing the role of schools and the goals they can realize if they choose to do so.

The Educator's Role in Facilitating Social Skills Development

Unfortunately, the responsibility educators have in relation to the instruction of social skills is vague. The curricula issued by Departments of Education are generally ambiguous in relation to what is expected of teachers. In their preservice training, teachers learn about discipline and how to control student behaviour which is disruptive to instruction but rarely are such topics as peer rejection, social acceptance of students with disabilities, or encouraging the participation of students who are shy, included in the course of studies for aspiring teachers. Nonetheless, many aspects of social skills programming (e.g., dealing with disruptive students) are part of the "hidden curriculum" or values which schools unconsciously teach and which consume significant proportions of educators time and energy each day in the classroom. Without appropriate social skills, students may not be able to either accept or benefit from academic instruction.

What then is the responsibility of educators to facilitate social skills development in the school environment? Perhaps the role can best be summarized in one statement. Real teachers teach social skills! Because a student's capacity to learn in a group situation (i.e., the social environment of today's classrooms) cannot be separated from the social competence required to interact effectively within this environment, teachers must teach social skills. Just as educators assume responsibility for the instruction of reading and the remediation of reading difficulties so they must assume responsibility for teaching the social skills which facilitate learning. For students who experience difficulty incorporating socially appropriate behaviour in the learning environment, remediation must be initiated. The following considerations support the inclusion of social skills instruction as a compulsory part of every teacher's role.

1. Many children do not spontaneously learn the social skills which are prerequisite to effective interaction with and social acceptance by their peer group. In Section I of this book, the implications a visual impairment might have upon the spontaneous acquisition of social skills were discussed. It was concluded that children with a visual impairment require formal instruction to learn the social skills essential to positive social interaction and peer acceptance. There are other students in every classroom who are known to have difficulty with the incidental learning of age appropriate social skills. Some students with learning disabilities may misinterpret or fail to respond to social cues which guide their peers in the development of prosocial behaviour. Youngsters who are gifted may sometimes experience difficulties understanding the interests and perceptions of children who are the same age. Other children, because of physical or emotional differences (e.g., obesity or shyness) may be stigmatized and rejected by their peers. In short, all classrooms usually have several children who are

at risk of being socially rejected or neglected by their peers (MacCuspie, 1991). The implementation of formal social skills training programs would ensure all children are exposed to skills which have significant long-term benefits (e.g., conflict resolution) as well as identifying and assisting those students who require specific and ongoing assistance in the area of social development.

2. Rejection by one's peers during the elementary school years is highly correlated with behaviour and/or emotional problems in both the teenage and adult years (Hartup, 1984; Parker & Asher, 1987). The establishment of positive relationships with both peers and adults is correlated with a child's level of social competence or mastery of social skills. As children begin to spend increasingly greater amounts of time interacting with peers than with adults, acceptance by the group becomes increasingly important and requires the addition and cultivation of new social skills and concepts. Factors associated with popularity among elementary school children were discussed in Chapter 2. It was noted that the crucial element in popularity during the elementary years is how a child behaves toward peers. Children who are gregarious, not critical, and who display an interest in their peers are observed to be those sought out by others. Such behaviours are inextricably linked with the mastery of social skills such as initiating interaction with others, recognizing the feelings of others, expressing an interest in others, negotiating and sharing. These are skills which can be taught and practised during routine classroom instruction.
3. Friendship is the source of stimulation for both social and intellectual development. Since friendship also provides an accepting relationship in which to refine social skills, children who do not have the social skills required to establish such relationships miss both the enjoyment friendship provides and invaluable learning inherent to this intimate relationship (e.g., perspective taking, moral development, concepts of justice).
4. Self-esteem, that is, how we feel about ourselves, evolves partly in response to reflections from others. If interaction with others is predominately positive, peer acceptance increases the likelihood that a student will have positive self-esteem. On the other hand, a student who is routinely ignored or rejected by peers frequently interprets this rejection as evidence of inadequacy or inferiority. Younger and more immature children are more strongly influenced by reflection from others in judging their own social competence than are adolescents (Tuttle, 1984). Therefore, it is crucial that social skills instruction begins early so that teachers can increase the probability that positive interaction with peers will promote the development of a positive self-esteem. When children enter school they become part of a world which is dominated by peer rather than adult interaction, thus their peers have a significant influence upon how they feel about themselves and the status of their abilities. Recent research on school drop-outs reports low self-esteem to be highly correlated with those who do not complete their schooling (Neufeld & Stevens, 1992). Educators must make

every attempt to orchestrate peer interaction which promotes the development of high self-esteem and increases the likelihood that all students will benefit from the time they spend in school.

5. The amount of time available to children to interact with their peers in school is remarkable. It appears that the major part of the school day is conducive to social exchange among children. Because students with inadequate social skills will miss many of the social and intellectual benefits available during these routine daily activities, teachers must intervene to facilitate social skills development during school hours. Schools are the only location where all children and youth spend a significant part of their growing years in the presence of their peers.
6. Teachers reap long-term benefits from instructing students in social skills because many of these skills contribute to the enhancement of the learning environment in the classroom. For example, students who have learned and who practice the social skills essential to group learning (e.g., seeking opinions, dignifying the errors of others, staying on task, following directions) require minimal intervention from teachers. Significant reductions in the amount of time the teacher must spend addressing disruptive behaviour or settling disputes among group members allows the teacher to focus on facilitating student learning. Furthermore, when teachers are perceived to accept the inappropriate social behaviour of some classmates (e.g., students who dominate discussions or who ridicule others), students interpret this action as one of condoning the behaviour. The recent concern for the sexual harassment of female students in our schools is further evidence that educators cannot overlook or minimize their responsibility in facilitating the development of social skills and setting standards for acceptable interaction among students.
7. Parents traditionally have been considered responsible for facilitating social skills development for their children and should continue to be intimately involved in this process after their child enters school. However, parents are not routinely available to observe and assist their children in the school setting. Interaction with school peers provides the primary source of exploration, experimentation and practice of social skills available to children. As well, they spend a significant part of their time in school during the period of their lives when they are developing and refining their social skills. Thus, schools provide both the natural setting and the opportunity to facilitate social skills development and teachers are the adults providing guidance in this environment.
8. Educators frequently feel empathetic yet helpless in dealing with a student who is observed to have difficulty acquiring and using appropriate social skills. Yet, educators do have the basic training and experiences prerequisite to the formal instruction of social skills. They have an understanding of child development and learning theory; experience in lesson planning, writing goals and objectives, evaluating student performance and initiating remediation based on evaluation; and experience with children within

a given age group and a specific setting upon which to base their evaluation of a student's social competence. With some initial training and familiarization with curriculum materials to augment their preservice training and classroom experience, most educators feel competent to teach social skills.

9. A child's social development does not occur in isolation of her/his cognitive or physical development. Educators cannot ignore the relationship between a student's potential to learn and the necessity of social skills which facilitate learning. During the school years children are experiencing ongoing changes in all aspects of their development. Those who demonstrate effective social skills while encountering such changes are advantaged students. The results of research have demonstrated the importance of "child-centred" learning and instruction which is relevant to the "whole child." Learning social skills which promote positive social interaction and contribute to a beneficial school experience must be considered compulsory.

All educators have a general responsibility to facilitate their students' development of social competence. They act as role models who promote the development of positive social relationships. Some educators may need training to develop skills in dealing effectively with the confrontational and defensive responses many students bring to the classroom or in strategies and methods used in teaching social skills. For some students, such as those with a visual impairment, formal instruction in social skills must never be left to chance. Research has documented the need for specific instruction in the development of social skills to be an essential part of programming for children with a visual impairment (MacCuspie, 1991; Sacks, Kekelis, & Gaylord Ross, 1992).

Students with Disabilities in Addition to a Visual Impairment

The number of children with one or more impairments in addition to a visual impairment has increased over the past several decades (Kirchner, 1990; Robinson, Jan & Kinnis, 1987). Agencies which have originated to provide services for those with a visual impairment, such as the Canadian National Institute for the Blind, have reported significant increases in the number of clients with disabilities in addition to a visual impairment. For the age group from birth through adolescence, it is estimated that fifty per cent of the group have at least one additional impairment.

Several factors are believed to have contributed to this change in the make-up of the population who are visually impaired (Gates, 1985). Improvements in medical science and an increased accessibility to the resulting advancements in life saving practices and technology have ensured the survival of infants who, in the past, would have died within a few days of their birth. Factors related to the actual cause of the visual impairment (i.e., etiological factors) have also played a significant role. Some conditions such as maternal rubella or retinopathy of prematurity frequently result in the child having several impairments (e.g., cognitive, hearing and visual impairments). Another factor which has contributed to the change in the makeup of the population with a visual impairment is the increased accessibility to programs and educational opportunities for children with disabilities. With the closing of custodial institutions and the passage of laws requiring formal educational placements for children with multiple disabilities, children who were once ineligible for schooling are now being enrolled. Many of these children have visual impairments. A final contributing factor is the improvement in and access to educational and clinical assessment. With general improvement in the identification and diagnosis of learning problems, greater numbers of children will have learning difficulties identified early in their educational years.

What Is Meant by Multiple Disabilities?

The term multiple disabilities is not one which has a consistent interpretation across North America. In the past, the term multihandicapped was typically used to describe individuals who had cognitive impairments in addition to one or more other disabilities (e.g., blindness, orthopaedic impairment). The Association for Persons with Severe Handicaps (TASH) identifies those with multiple disabilities as:

> *individuals of all ages who require extensive ongoing support in more than one major life activity in order to participate in integrated community settings and to enjoy a quality of life that is available to citizens with fewer or no disabilities. Support may be required for life activities such as mobility, communication, self-care, and learning, as necessary for independent living, employment, and self-sufficiency (Lindley, 1990, p.1)*

In the United States federal laws outline specific criteria to categorize various disabilities. An individual identified as having multiple disabilities has "concomitant impairments. . . the combination of which causes such severe educational problems that these learners cannot be accommodated in special education programs solely for one of the disabilities (Shea & Bauer, 1994, p. 240). In Canada federal laws relevant to educational labels, special education services and program requirements do not exist. Here, the provinces have jurisdiction over education and related laws, policies and procedures, terminology, and resources. Approaches can vary greatly from province to province. Frequently, terms similar to those used in the United States have been adopted but others have been devised specifically for a particular province or school board. A severe cognitive impairment is usually identified as one of the several disabilities of individuals who have multiple disabilities (Winzer, 1990). Since the term multiple disabilities provides limited information about a student's learning needs, it is essential to consider the particular disabilities or impairments a given learner may have, the severity of these impairments, and the implications they have for learning and performance in various situations.

Regardless of the definition of "multiple disabilities" adopted, families of children with additional impairments must address many issues — financial concerns associated with those who are medically fragile; concerns about the additional time and energy required to parent a child with multiple disabilities; care for their child when he/she reaches adulthood if ongoing supervision or assistance is apt to be necessary; and society's acceptance of a child who may be viewed as very different from other children. Educators are also presented with many new challenges when a student with multiple disabilities is enrolled in their school. There are questions about the type of educational programming to be provided, access to the specialists who are knowledgeable about the child's various impairments, provision of the appropriate materials and resources, and the inclusion of this student as a valued member of the student population. What must be recognized from the beginning, is the uniqueness of each individual. The strategies to promote social interaction and acceptance will need to be customized to enhance the strengths and talents of the particular individual and to address the specific environments in which the student will be functioning.

Students with a Second Impairment

The effect of two impairments (i.e., a visual impairment and a second impairment) upon development and learning is dependent upon both the nature of the second impairment and the extent to which it interferes with an already limited access to visual information. A child with a visual impairment and a physical disability (e.g., uses a wheelchair for mobility) would probably experience unique challenges associated with social interaction within the pupil culture. In some situations, the student might not be able to participate in the same activities as peers (e.g., playing soccer at recess) while in other circumstances, opportunities to participate might be influenced by such things as the accessibility of parts of the school and the playground for students in a wheelchair. The complexity of the multiple factors effecting the social integration of a student with both a visual and a physical impairment would be compounded because of the considerations relevant to each impairment.

It is essential that all programming plans to enhance social integration include a thorough examination of the effects of the second impairment upon social interaction, development and learning. The findings of research on children with specific disabilities provides important information for consideration by the collaborative team (i.e., parents, teachers, special educators, medical professionals, and administrators). In considering children with learning disabilities, for example, Andrews and Lupart (1993) outlined the findings of research examining social ability. Children with learning disabilities were reported to be:

> *(1) less proficient than nonlearning-disabled children in taking another person's point of view during interpersonal situations; (2) more egocentric (unable to understand the feelings and positions of*

> *others, and to adjust to the different needs of their listeners); and (3) unable to function efficiently in both speaker and listener roles, particularly in their inability to provide sufficient information for communication to be adequately shared and understood. (p. 549)*

Given what is known about the implications of a visual impairment upon social interaction, it is apparent that the addition of a learning disability could have significant implications for the social integration of the student with such a combination of impairments. Not only will the child have difficulty accessing visual information but, in all probability, will also struggle with the appropriate interpretation of the information which is received.

Although research findings do not necessarily identify which impairments are most detrimental to social interaction, it seems probable that some impairments may pose a greater degree of difficulty relative to social integration than others. Therefore, the degree to which a combination of impairments may interfere with social interaction and acceptance by peers needs to be assessed in relation to the specific implications the particular impairments create and the social context in which they are examined. Consider the profound effects of a dual sensory loss such as blindness and deafness upon communication. A child with this combination of impairments is virtually isolated from all but a few highly trained interpreters who must act as the messenger for both the child and those with whom he/she wishes to communicate. Obviously, a dual sensory loss such as deafness and blindness would require different approaches to learning, social skills training, and social environmental adaptations than would be recommended for a child with a visual impairment and a learning disability.

Social Relationships of Individuals with Multiple Disabilities

The effect of multiple disabilities upon development and learning is not only a combination or aggregate of the impact of the various impairments but a complex compounding of factors which are frequently difficult to anticipate and assess. Being aware of the serious implications vision loss can have on the spontaneous development of social relationships, what then might be the implications for these children if they also have cognitive, hearing and physical impairments? The need to receive input from a number of specialists to plan for the social integration of a child with multiple disabilities is critical to understanding the barriers to communication and learning for this student. Specialists such as physiotherapists and speech pathologists need to provide input as to how the child's physical needs and communication can be addressed in the integrated setting. The teacher of the visually impaired must consider the suggestions of other professionals relative to access to visual information and necessary adaptations to curriculum materials or programs. Of course, observations and insights from the classroom teacher, parents and administrator must guide the basic direction of the integration plan.

It is not uncommon, particularly for educators involved with children with special needs, to know of a student who appeared to have severe learning difficulties or problematic behaviours but with timely and insightful intervention was able to make significant, even inconceivable progress. Consider the achievements of Helen Keller who despite the loss of both vision and hearing was a writer, lecturer and advocate for those with disabilities. Her accomplishments stand as an example of what may be possible when the appropriate teaching strategies and a supportive social environment are provided.

In our culture today, social patterns among both children and adults tend to be characterized by relationships between those who are similar. Friends, or those with whom one chooses to spend time, most often share similar interests, are of comparable intellectual ability, and are of the same gender. People seem to be both attracted to and comfortable in the presence of those who are like them. In short, one's friendship relationships tend to be highly homogeneous. Voeltz (1984) suggested that the integration of individuals with multiple disabilities provided opportunities for society to experience a new type of friendship:

> *Surely it is possible to value and experience mutually rewarding, "heterogeneous" friendships—with people who are somehow quite different from our usual friends. Heterogeneous interactions among individuals and cultures most probably represent a higher stage in social development than do segregation, rejection, and isolation from one another. (p. 180)*

The nature of friendships between those with and without disabilities has frequently been a serious concern of both teachers and parents. All too frequently within integrated classroom situations, social interactions among children with multiple disabilities and their peers are uni-directional relationships. That is, the child with multiple disabilities is viewed as the recipient of altruistically motivated attention from peers who do not have disabilities. Frequently the child with multiple disabilities is the passive recipient of verbal comments, often spoken in an immature intonation; assistance with activities such as moving from place to place; help with daily living skills such as dressing, or support to participate in routine learning activities. In such a scenario, the individual with multiple disabilities may seem to be the recipient of the charitable efforts of sympathetic peers rather than a valued contributing member of the class. Social interactions between children with disabilities and their peers must be mutually beneficial if they are to be lasting relationships. The intention of such relationships is to provide increased skills in social interaction for both individuals. "Learning how to interact with severely handicapped persons not only implies the development of new social and communication skills, but also provides practice in adapting behaviour to widely varying social demands (Voeltz, 1984, p. 180). Children without disabilities who master the social skills necessary to communicate appropriately and spontaneously with individuals with multiple disabilities are the beneficiaries of a capability which will serve them well throughout their lives and will make a significant contribution toward the realization of a truly inclusive society.

Programming to Promote Social Integration of Students with Multiple Disabilities

Chapter 7 provided suggestions to enhance the social interaction and acceptance of students with a visual impairment. Most of this information is appropriate for all children with a visual impairment, regardless of the presence of additional disabilities. However, children who are visually impaired in addition to other severe or profound disabilities may benefit from intervention focused primarily upon their inclusion in the school. Since the advocacy for integration of individuals with severe and profound disabilities began in Canada in the 1970s, considerable effort has been focused on the meaningful inclusion of children with multiple disabilities in both their schools and communities. A planning approach known as the McGill Action Planning System (MAPS) designed by Marsha Forest and Judith Snow of the Canadian Association for Community Living has become widely used in many parts of Canada (Forest, Vandercook, & York, 1989).

The MAPS Process

MAPS is a future oriented and team-building planning strategy. It is based on the belief that the needs of students with severe and profound disabilities are best met in the classroom with age-appropriate peers and that building friendships and mutually supportive relationships are at the heart of personal growth, learning and quality of life. Using the natural classroom setting and everyday classroom activities as opportunities to incorporate learning activities for the student with multiple disabilities, MAPS requires the routine input of classmates in devising effective ways to include the student. The imaginative problem-solving abilities of both adults and children who care about the student are used to design learning activities and opportunities for meaningful participation for the student with multiple disabilities. Most importantly, MAPS recognizes the expertise of parents in program planning and acknowledges that they have the most at stake in the development and well-being of their child. Given this recognition, MAPS empowers parents to become key decision makers on the planning team.

The MAPS process is usually initiated after the student with multiple disabilities has been in the regular classroom for several months and is well known to classmates. The goal of the MAPS process is not only to create a support network for the student with multiple disabilities but also to establish a team committed to working to realize the inclusion of the student in school life. A team meeting attended by parents, regular and special education personnel, and several classmates of the student is the first step in the process. A facilitator guides the participants through their consideration of seven key questions designed to gather information and to provide the basis for program development. The seven key questions are outlined below.

1. **What is the individual's history?**

Family members of the student with multiple disabilities are asked to outline the key milestones in the student's life. They share information about such things as the cause of the disability, the types of programs in which the child has participated, and the important events in the child's life.

2. **What is your dream for the individual?**

Participants are encouraged to think about and articulate the future they would like for the student with multiple disabilities. This question forces the team to think about the direction in which the student is heading and what will need to happen if their vision is to become a reality. Future residential accommodations and opportunities for involvement in the community are frequently identified during this discussion. With a shared vision to guide team members, the current barriers and attitudes which detract from the expectations for students with multiple disabilities can be eliminated.

3. **What is your nightmare for the individual?**

This questions offers team members an opportunity to verbalize their fears for the student's future. Parents frequently talk about their fears of the child being left alone or institutionalized when they are no longer available to provide the necessary care.

4. **Who is the individual?**

Everyone on the team offer words to describe the student with multiple disabilities from their perspectives (e.g., classmate, brother, sister, daughter, neighbour). In describing the student with multiple disabilities as "comical," a sibling can assist other participants to view the student in many different ways. The purpose is to create an image of the "whole individual" for the team.

5. **What are the individual's strengths, interests, and abilities?**

The identification of the student's positive characteristics is intended to provide the basis for program planning. By identifying such things as interests, potential sources of motivation for the student's participation in various activities can be identified. This question also serves to increase the awareness of team members since different participants bring perspectives from different situations (e.g., classroom, playground, home).

6. **What are the individual's needs?**

Each team member identifies the student's needs from her/his perspective. Teachers may identify skills to be mastered while parents might outline opportunities for social interaction with peers. These needs are then prioritized by the group and identified for incorporation in program planning.

7. **What should the individual's ideal school day look like and what must be done to make it happen?**

The schedule for a classmate in the regular class is usually used as a basis upon which to plan the activities for the student with multiple disabilities. For example, the physical education period is an ideal time to complete the exercise routine outlined by the physiotherapist. The team develops strategies which enhance the full integration of the student with peers while addressing the individual learning needs of the student. The supports and resources needed to implement the plan are also identified.

After the seven questions have been considered by the team, an opportunity is provided for members to respond to their feelings about the process. Participant feedback is welcomed and accepted. Next, the team prioritizes actions to be initiated, identifies specific roles for those involved in implementing the program, and confirms timelines for program implementation, monitoring and evaluation.

For students at the secondary level, MAPS is modified both in its program focus and in the composition of the planning team. Programming for a secondary student involves not only inclusion in the classroom but also in various locations in the community (e.g., stores, work sites). As the student nears the age when school involvement will be completed, a focus on transition into the community is required. From a logistical perspective, the MAPS process for secondary students varies because of the way secondary schools are departmentalized. Since the student has many teachers with different classmates in most classes, participants on the team are chosen based on different criteria than those used in the elementary school setting. Teachers are chosen contingent on their interest and anticipated future involvement with the student. Classmates who express an interest in being involved, know the student, or are a neighbourhood peer of the student are usually good team members at the secondary level. Community members may also become part of the planning team at this level. Given the programmatic and logistical differences between the MAPS for elementary and secondary students, the focus of both is the inclusion of the individuals with multiple disabilities in the ordinary life activities of their peers.

MAPS is an affirmative process that utilizes the collective resources of classmates, family members, neighbours, friends and educators to plan for the inclusion in school and community of a student with multiple disabilities. Becoming part of a school or community cannot be decreed and there is not one standard approach or strategy for every individual. Inclusion is a social process and planning systems such as MAPS are important because they provide a vision distinguished by schools that welcome diversity among its members.

The Role of The Teacher Assistant in Enhancing Inclusion

The use of paraprofessionals (i.e., those who do not have formal training as teachers) to assist in the education of students with disabilities has increased dramatically with the move to integrated placements for these students (New

Brunswick, 1994). When a student is not able to self-initiate participation in classroom activities or when his/her behaviour is frequently disruptive to the learning environment, a teacher assistant is usually hired.

The responsibilities assigned paraprofessionals in the integrated setting are as numerous as the titles by which they have become identified (e.g., teacher assistant, student aide, classroom helper). For the purpose of this discussion, the term teacher assistant will be used in reference to the member of the educational support staff who is assigned to assist with students who have special learning needs. It is critical that the roles and responsibilities of these staff members are clearly defined. In New Brunswick the responsibilities of a teacher assistant are outlined as follows.

> *This is work of limited complexity primarily in assisting teachers in the performance of their duties. Work is under the supervision of a teacher and involves providing assistance to individuals and groups of students. Work includes providing assistance in classrooms, libraries, shops and laboratories; assisting in supervision of students; assisting with the preparation of teaching aids and the assembly of materials as directed by the teacher; assisting in maintaining records, and generally assisting teachers in functions designed to fulfill the instructional, social and/or behavioral goals and objectives as planned by the teacher; performing various other general support duties, and assisting with the physical needs of exceptional students. (New Brunswick Department of Education, 1994, p. iv)*

Because the role assigned to a teacher assistant can have a significant influence on the social acceptance and inclusion of students with a disability, the responsibility of this staff member is of considerable importance to the collaborative team involved in planning for the integration of these students.

The initial intention of administrators in providing teacher assistants for students with a disability was both to address the special needs of the student and to provide the classroom teacher with help in accommodating the demands of the class, in general. However, as integration has been implemented in schools the nature of the teacher assistant role has been modified and varied to address not only the special needs of the students but also the instructional style of teachers, the demands of parents, and the administrative approach of the principal or school district supervisors. The valuable role of the teacher assistant in the integration process is attested to by educators. Unfortunately, the position can be misused in two ways which are extremely detrimental to students. First, there is the practice of assigning the teacher assistant to the student rather than to the class as a whole. The student relies on the teacher assistant to provide access to the educational environment. When a teacher assistant is assigned to a particular student an interdependence develops between them — the student relies on the teacher assistant to involve her/him in the school program while the teacher assistant is employed as long as the student requires assistance. Because a teacher assistant and a student may be together for several years, a special bond frequently develops between them. The danger in this relationship is the potential for the student to become overly dependent upon the teacher assistant and fail to develop the independence he/she may be capable of acquiring. The teacher assistant, on the other hand, may perceive the success of the student as an explicit statement of his/her competence as a staff member. When students are assigned homework or required to complete tests, the teacher assistant may feel a personal responsibility for the completion of the student's work or the level of performance. Classmates of a student with a disability are usually very aware of the assistance provided this student in the regular classroom. Those privileges provided the student which are perceived to provide an unfair advantage to this student are frequently resented by classmates. This resentment can be particularly intense if the learning environment is a very competitive one and may often result in classmates ignoring or rejecting the student with a disability.

Another problem associated with the assignment of a teacher assistant to a specific student is related to the significant amount of time the assistant may spend with the student with a disability. Extended periods of time in direct association with the student may act to interfere with the spontaneous social interaction which typically occurs when children are not involved in classroom work or during scheduled breaks such as recess. At certain ages (e.g., early adolescence) the presence of any adult during "free time" in school is considered to be an intrusion. As well, classmates may feel the student is content in the company of the teacher assistant or has little interest in pursuing interaction with peers. When a student is given unlimited attention by the teacher assistant, peers may perceive the student to be unable to function independently. Therefore, the teacher assistant must be acutely aware of her/his potential to act as a barrier to social interaction between the student with a disability and classmates, to foster myths associated with the helplessness of those with disabilities, and to contribute to the student's preference to affiliate with adults.

The second issue associated with the misuse of the teacher assistant position is the practice of assigning this staff member the instructional responsibilities of a teacher. Such a practice devalues students who are disabled since it implies that they do not warrant or cannot benefit from the instruction of the "real" teacher in the classroom. In addition, assignment of teacher assistant to a student significantly reduces the contact the classroom teacher has with this student and hence, decreases the likelihood that her/his instructional expertise will be used to assess the student's learning strengths and needs. When examining the implications this practice may have on the social integration of the student, it is evident that a student being instructed by the teacher assistant, often in an isolated part of the classroom, is not an integral part of the class. Furthermore, teachers who have limited interaction with students with a disability in the classroom cannot model the positive acceptance of difference for classmates nor can they develop essential skills in working with students with a range of learning styles and needs. In summary, the practice of assigning instructional responsibilities to a teacher assistant is irresponsible from both an educational and ethical standpoint. Educators and parents need to be alert to the potential barriers to social acceptance which may be correlated with the responsibilities assigned the teacher assistant but they must also capitalize on the significant role this staff member can play in enhancing the social acceptance and interaction of the student with a disability. Teacher assistants usually have a wealth of experience with students with a disability and can make valuable contributions as members of the collaborative school team. As teacher assistants, they have many opportunities to observe the social acceptance and interaction of the student and to record situations which require modification to enhance the participation and learning of the student. In many cases, as mentioned previously, the teacher assistant has been with the same student for more than a year and has tremendous insight into both the affective and intellectual development of the student. More importantly, the teacher assistant who has developed a trusting relationship with the student can provide the encouragement and support the student needs to take the daily risks inherent in striving for inclusion in a world designed by and for those without disabilities.

Organizing Inclusive Playgrounds

Elementary school playgrounds hold tremendous potential as the locations where social integration can be exemplified. Play is the natural medium for interaction among children. "Children experience their humanness and what it means to be a social being, through play" (McGill, 1984, p. 4). Play provides opportunities to develop physical fitness and motor coordination, to expand the imagination, to focus attention and concentration, to explore and manipulate the environment, and to practice and refine social skills and interpersonal communication in a non-threatening environment. For children, play is a voluntary activity that affords the freedom to interact with friends and the opportunity to just have fun.

Similar to many other children with a disability, children with a visual impairment may have limited opportunities to play. The child may be limited by his/her level of physical agility or a delayed development of actual play skills. The amount of time available for play is often restricted because of the extra time it takes these children to complete routine classroom activities or those associated with daily living skills such as independently dressing to go outside for recess. In addition to the regular education curriculum, children with a visual impairment have time available to learn disability specific skills such as orientation and mobility or use of adaptive technology. Although both educators and parents acknowledge the value of play in the healthy development of children, many underestimate the detrimental consequences endured by children who have limited opportunities to play. For a child with a severe visual impairment, the absence of play can have particularly devastating results. Poor physical fitness, posture and gait; preference for passive or self-stimulating behaviours; and a tendency to be self-centred and inept in interpersonal communication are characteristics frequently reported in relation to children who are visually impaired and who have not developed appropriate play skills. These children experience difficulties with play early in life when they do not receive the visual information which motivates sighted children to explore their environments and imitate the actions of others. Knowing the significant physical, cognitive and social benefits of play, the importance of organizing meaningful play opportunities for children who are visually impaired cannot be overlooked.

There are two issues which need to be addressed when considering how to orchestrate play opportunities for children with a visual impairment in the school setting. First, play activities need to be structured, at least initially, to ensure the active participation of the child who is visually impaired. Many of the factors which exclude this child from the routine activities on school playgrounds were discussed in Section II. In planning for meaningful participation, organizers need to ensure that the child with a visual impairment has timely access to visual information, adaptations implemented to ensure full involvement, and a level of skill which allows the child to enjoy the activity.

The second issue is associated with the nature of play which frequently characterizes elementary school playgrounds. Some researchers have reported that children's games are too competitive, violent and aggressive (McGill, 1984). Games which result in fear of failure, rejection by peers or hurt feelings do not belong on school playgrounds where children are basically held captive for specific periods of time each school day. The competitive attitude reflected in society is another source of negative influence upon the games of children (Orlick, 1978). When games involve a "win-lose" component or a "win at all costs" outlook, many children are losers, including those who are visually impaired. Educators and parents promoting the inclusion of all children in our schools need to implement structured play opportunities which allow children to develop appropriate play skills and cooperative play activities which welcome all participants regardless of level of competence.

Cooperative Games on the Playground

McGill (1984) has been involved in promoting integrated play and recreational opportunities for individuals with intellectual disabilities for many years. When analyzing play opportunities for children, McGill insisted that:

> *In order to facilitate integration, it is important that play providers be able to create an accepting and supportive environment where children feel free to interact and to play with one another. The environment should be one where all children, regardless of their skill level, are encouraged to participate to the best of their ability. It should be an environment that is fun and motivating and that permits each child to develop within his or her own growth and development patterns. The environment should not be one that puts undue stress on skill level or on negatively-valued differences. (p. 3)*

A Canadian professor named Terry Orlick became involved with the philosophy of cooperative games developed in ancient cultures. Through his study of play he became concerned about the relationship between the existence of few alternatives to competitive games available in present day educational and recreational settings and the resulting high percentage of teenagers who dropped out of competitive sports and became physically inactive. Orlick became interested in investigating alternative play structures and opportunities which would be accessible to all children. Cooperative games which focus on developing a positive sense of self and others provided Orlick his means of addressing what he had concluded was an increasing "problem of inactivity and 'spectatoritis'" (McGill, 1984, p. 2). Orlick felt strongly about the need to nurture opportunities for positive social interaction as a means to making physical activity a motivational pursuit.

Orlick (1978) outlined four basic components to cooperative games. The first was cooperation. Games were designed so that they required communication, interaction and cooperation by compelling the participants to work together and to help one another to achieve a common goal. The second component was fun. In cooperative games this essential component was intensified because the participants were free to play with one another and not against one another, hence, removing the stress of failure. Acceptance was the third component of cooperative games and was nurtured by ensuring each player had a meaningful role to play. The fourth component was involvement which resulted as a consequence of having had an opportunity to belong to the group and make a contribution to achieving the goal of the game. Orlick (1978a) also outlined four specific structures which could be used in playing cooperative games. There were cooperative games with no losers in which a group shared a common goal (e.g., to trap a large mountain of air under a parachute held by the players); cooperative score games which were devised so that each group or team worked to amass one collective score; reversal games in which participants were routinely rotated between teams or reverse scoring where points went to the other team with the objective being to assist the other team in scoring; and semi-cooperative games in which teams played against each other but every participant was given an equal opportunity to play and the importance of the score was de-emphasized. By implementing Orlick's four basic components and specific cooperative game structures, play providers have had tremendous success in creating inclusive play activities.

Implementing Cooperative Games on the Playground

Although time spent on the playground in elementary schools usually involves limited adult intervention, implementing cooperative games will require an adult or older student to take control and lead the games. Cooperative games are easily adapted to specific age levels or to meet a particular student's level of skill and ability (McGill, 1984). Participants are encouraged to work together as partners and to assist other members to both participate in and enjoy the game. Since cooperative games are taught mainly through demonstration and performance, children learn them easily. The leader must attend to structuring opportunities for positive interaction and monitoring the accessibility of the game to those children with disabilities.

The collaborative team formed to promote the social and instructional integration of the student with a visual impairment will need to consider their options for providing cooperative games on the playground. Volunteers may be trained and assigned to lead cooperative games on the playground. Teachers assigned to playground supervision or playground supervisors may also be able to take on the responsibility for having cooperative games running in one area of the playground. The physical education teacher may become the resource person with an array of creative ideas in providing cooperative playground activities. With the introduction of different games, it is possible that over time the students themselves will develop the level of skill to independently run the games and adults can gracefully bow out to monitor the social interaction on the playground from a distance. The benefits children will enjoy in active and meaningful participation on the playground will be evident both in the classroom and in the community.

The provision for participation in cooperative games should not be the only solution for elementary school age students who are visually impaired. Many of the playground activities which are popular at a given time of the school year can be adapted to ensure the meaningful participation of the student with a visual impairment. Balls with auditory output, tees for holding balls in position for batting, playground equipment with many spaces for climbing and exploring, sandboxes with defined spaces, and embossed or highlighted hopscotch patterns are but a few of the options which can be provided to enhance the participation of a child with a visual impairment. Many seasonal activities, such as coasting, are accessible without major adaptations if classmates are knowledgeable about the need for their classmate with a visual impairment to be actively involved and if they understand the implications of this impairment on participation on the playground. Creative solutions come with knowledge!

Conclusion

"Change is in the wind." Educators have been expected to make significant changes in both their educational philosophies and practices during the past few decades. Looking back, it is apparent that the underlying beliefs that maintained the philosophies of thirty years ago and guided the instructional practices of students with a visual impairment have proven to be flawed. Children who are visually impaired can be educated in their neighbourhood schools. Their parents can provide the support and instruction essential to the development of independence and positive self-esteem. Their classmates can be made aware of the implications of a visual impairment on social interaction and their schools can create a social environment which enhances both the academic progress and the social acceptance of students. These things have been accomplished by open-minded individuals with a problem-solving approach to the challenges integration of students with a disability have posed.

The controversial issues discussed in this chapter are only an example of the many which will continue to arise as educators and parents examine and learn from experiences with integration. Advocates for inclusive schools have identified major changes required throughout the education system (e.g., school-based inclusive teaming, an emphasis on sharing professional expertise, curricular restructuring to prepare students for the 21st century). Success in dealing with proposed changes will be realized if participants are able to openly discuss and analyze the implications, merits, complications, and long-range effects of reorganization. Although at times it may seem to be an overwhelming challenge, one must remember "we already have the technical and psychological knowledge to do what needs to be done to make school a positive experience for children. What we need to do is decide when, if, and how we will do it.

Appendix A

References for Cooperative Learning

Andrini, B. (1989). *Cooperative learning and mathematics: A multi-structural approach.* San Juan Capistrano, CA: Resources for Teachers.

Bennett, B., Rolheiser-Bennett, C., & Stevahn, L. (1991). *Cooperative learning: Where heart meets mind*. Toronto, ONT: Educational Connections.

Bina, M.J. (1986). Social skills development through cooperative group learning strategies. *Education of the Visually Handicapped, 18*(1), 27-40.

Clarke, J., Wideman, R., & Eadie, S. (1990). *Together we learn*. Scarborough, ONT: Prentice-Hall.

Curran, L. (1990). *Cooperative learning lessons for little* ones: Literature-based language arts and social skills. San Juan Capistrano, CA: Resources for Teachers.

Davidson, N. (Ed.). (1989). *Cooperative learning in* mathematics: A handbook for teachers. Reading, MA: Addison-Wesley.

Holm, A., Schultz, D., Winget, P., & Wurzbach, L. (1987). *Cooperative activities for the home: Parents working with* teachers to support cooperative learning. Sacramento, CA: Resources in Special Education.

Johnson, D.W. & Johnson, R.T. (1989). *Leading the cooperative school*. Edina, MN: Interaction Book.

Johnson, D.W., Johnson, R.T. & Holubec, E.J. (1987). *Structuring cooperative learning: Lesson plans for teachers*. Edina, MN: Interaction Book.

Johnson, D.W., Johnson, R.T. & Holubec, E.J. (1990). *Circles of learning: Cooperation in the classroom*. Edina, MN: Interaction Book.

Johnson, D.W., Johnson, R.T. & Holubec, E.J. (1991). *Cooperation in the classroom*. Edina, MN: Interactio n Book.

Johnson, R.T., & Johnson, D.W. (1981). Building friendships between handicapped and non-handicapped children: Effects of cooperative and individualistic instruction. *American Educational Research Journal, 18*, 415-423.

Johnson, R.T., & Johnson, D.W. (1984). Classroom learning structure and attitudes toward handicapped students in mainstream settings: A theoretical model and research evidence. In R.L. Jones (Ed.), *Attitudes and attitude change in special education: Theory and practice*. Reston, VA: Council for Exceptional Children.

Kohn, A. (1991). Don't spoil the promise of cooperative learning. *Educational Leadership, 48*(5), 93-94.

Male, M., Johnson, R., Johnson, D., & Anderson, M. (1988). *Cooperative learning and computers: An activity guide for teachers*. Santa Cruz, CA: Educational Applecations.

McCabe, M.E., & Rhodes, J. (1988). *The nurturing classroom. Developing self-esteem, thinking skills and responsibility through simple cooperation*. Willits, CA: ITA Publications.

McGill, J. (1984). *Play for play's sake: Cooperative games as a strategy for integration*. Downsview, ONT: Canadian Association for Community Living.

Ontario Secondary School Teachers' Federation. (1989). *Independent learning: Process to product*. Toronto, ONT.

Orlick, T. (1978). *The cooperative sports and games book*. New York: Pantheon.

Orlick, T. (1981). *The second cooperative sports and games book*. New York: Pantheon.

Schwartz, S., & Pollishuke, M. (1990). *Creating the child-centred classroom*. Concord, ONT: Irwin.

Sharan, Y., & Sharan, S. (1990). *Cooperative learning: Theory and research*. Westport, CT: Praeger.

Slavin, R.E. (1986) *Using student team learning*. Baltimore, MD: The Johns Hopkins Team Learning Project.

Slavin, R.E. (1989). *Cooperative learning. Theory, research, and practice*. Englewood Cliffs, NJ: Prentice-Hall.

Slavin, R.E. (1991). Synthesis of research on cooperative learning. *Educational Leadership, 48*(5), 71-82.

Stone, J.M. (1989). *Cooperative learning and language arts:* A multi-structural approach. San Juan Capistrano, CA: Resources for Teachers.

Appendix B

References for Social Skills Training

Asher, S.R., & Gottman, J. (Ed.). (1981). *The development of children's friendships*. New York: Cambridge University Press.

Asher, S.R., & Taylor, A.R. (1981). Social outcomes of mainstreaming: Sociometric assessment and beyond. *Exceptional Educational Quarterly, 1*(4), 13-30.

Asher, S.R., Hymel, S., & Renshaw, P.D. (1984). Loneliness in children. Childhood Development, 55, 1456-1464.

Bina, M.J. (1986). Social skills development through cooperative group learning strategies. *Education of the Visually Handicapped, 18*(1), 27-40.

Can Do! Video Series. *Making Friends: Social skills and play.* Louisville, KY, Visually Impaired Preschool Services, Inc.

CASE Research Committee. (1993). *Social skills instruction for students with disabilities.* Reston, VA: Council for Exceptional Children.

Gresham, F.M. (1983). Social skills assessment as a component of mainstreaming placement decisions. *Exceptional Children, 49*, 331-336.

Hoben, M. (1976). *Reducing Isolation in the Mainstream: Final Report.* Minneapolis: Hennepin Technical Centers.

Krenz, D. & MacDougall, D. (1984). *25 classroom activities to change the world through encouragement*. Edmonton, AL.

McConnell, S.R., & Odom, S.L. (1986). Sociometrics: Peer-referenced measures and the assessment of social competence. In P. S. Stain, M.J. Guralnick, & H.M. Walker (Eds.), Children's Social Behavior: Development, Assessment, and Modification. Orlando, FL: Academic Press.

Nezer, H., Nezer, B., & Siperstein, G. (1985). *Improving children's social skills: Techniques for teachers (Grant # DIF G5583016). Boston, MA: The Center for the Study of Social Acceptance, University of Massachusetts.*

Raver, S.A. & Drash, P.W. (1988). Increasing social skills training for visually impaired children. *Education of the Visually Handicapped, 19*, 147-155.

Read, L.F. (1989). An examination of the social skills of blind kindergarten children. *Education of the Visually Handicapped, 20*, 142-155.

Sacks, S., & Gaylord-Ross, R. (1989). Peer-mediated and teacher-directed social skills training for visually impaired students. *Behavior Therapy, 20*, 619-638.

Sacks, S., Kekelis, L.S. & Gaylord-Ross, R.J. (Eds.). (1992) *The development of social skills by blind and visually impaired students*. New York: American Foundation for the Blind.

Swallow, R. & Huebner, K.M. (1987). *How to thrive, not just survive: A guide to developing independent life skills for blind and visually impaired children and youth.* New York: American Foundation for the Blind.

Van Hasselt, V.B., Simon, J., & Mastantuono, A.K. (1982). Social skills training for blind children and adolescents. *Education of the Visually Handicapped, 14*(2), 34-39.

Sociometric Instruments

Agard, J.A., Veldman, D.J., Kaufman, M.J., & Semmel, M.I. *How I feel about others: An instrument of the PRIME Inventory Battery*. Project PRIME, Technical Report, undated.

Bailey, J.A., & Pierce, K.A. (1975). The friendship rating scale: A sociometric instrument. *Elementary School Guidance and Counseling, 9*, 218-225.

Coie, J.D., Dodge, K.A., & Coppotelli, H. (1982). Dimensions and types of social status: A cross-age *perspective. Developmental Psychology, 18*, 557-570.

Nezer, H., Nezer, B., & Siperstein, G. (1985). *Improving children's social skills: Techniques for teachers. Book of Activities* (Grant # DIE G5583016). Boston, MA: The Center for the Study of Social Acceptance, University of Massachusetts.

Shapiro, S.B., & Sobel, M. (1981). Two multinominal random sociometric voting models. *Journal of Educational Statistics, 6*, 287-310.

Social Skills Checklists

Goldstein, A.P., Sprafkin, R.P., Gershaw, J., & Klein, P. (1980). *Skillstreaming the adolescent: A structured learning approach to teaching prosocial skills*. Champaign, IL: Research Press.

Loumiet, R., & Levack, N. (1991). *Independent living: A curriculum with adaptations for students with visual impairments: Volume I: Social competence*. Austin, TX: Texas School for the Blind and Visually Impaired.

McGinnis, E., Goldstein, A.P., Sprafkin, R.P., & Gershaw, J. (1984). Skillstreaming the elementary child: *A guide for teaching prosocial skills*. Champaign, IL: Research Press.

Read, L.F. (1989). An examination of the social skills of blind kindergarten children. *Education of the VisuallyHandicapped, 20*, 142-155.

Stephens, T.M. (1980). *Social behavior assessment*. Columbus, OH: Cedar Press.

Social Skills Curricula

Camp, B.W. (1984). *Think aloud: Increasing social and cognitive skills. A problem solving program for children. Primary level*. Champaign, IL: Research Press.

Cheney, D., Morgan, D., & Young, R. (1985). *Assertiveness skills for adolescents*. Logan, UT: Utah State University.

Croft, N.B., & Robinson, L.W. (1976). *Project vision-up curriculum: A training program for preschool handicapped children*. Boise, ID: Educational Products Training Foundation.

Jackson, N. F. (1983) *Getting along with others: Teaching social effectiveness to children*. Champaign, IL: Research Press.

Jones, R.L., & Chiba, C. (1985). *Social skills assessment and intervention (Final Report)*. Bethesda, MD: National Institute of Child Health and Human Development.

Loumiet, R., & Levack, N. (1991). *Independent living: A curriculum with adaptations for students with visual impairments: Volume I: Social competence*. Austin, TX: Texas School for the Blind and Visually Impaired.

McCallum, B.J., & Sacks, S. (Eds.). (1994). *Social skills curriculum for children with visual impairments*. Santa Clara County, CA: SCORE Regionalization Project.

Nezer, H., Nezer, B., & Siperstein, G. (1985). *Improving children's social skills: Techniques for teachers* (Grant # DIE G5583016). Boston, MA: The Center for the Study of Social Acceptance, University of Massachusetts.

Peterson, T.J., Young, R., & Morgan, D.P. (1985). *Talking with others: Teaching conversation skills to children and adolescents*. Logan, UT: Utah State University.

Stephens, T.M. (1978). *Social skills in the classroom*. Columbus, OH: Cedar Press.

Transition (1979) *A Program to help students through the difficult passage from childhood to middle adolescence*. Circle Pines, MN: American Guidance Services.

Walker, L., McConnell, S., Holmes, D., Todis, B., Walker, L., & Golden, N. (1983). *The Walker social skills curriculum: The ACCEPTS program*. Austin, TX: Pro Ed.

Walker, H.M., Todis, B., Holmes, D., & Horton, G. (1988). *The Walker social skills curriculum: The ACCEPTS program*. Austin, TX: Pro Ed.

Young, R., Morgan, D., Likins, M., Cheney, D., & Peterson, T.J. (1984). *Basic social interaction preskills*. Logan, UT: Utah State University.

School/Classroom Climate Assessment Instruments

Nezer, H., Nezer, B., & Siperstein, G. (1985). *Improving children's social skills: Techniques for teachers. Book of Activities* (Grant # DIE G5583016). Boston, MA: The Center for the Study of Social Acceptance, University of Massachusetts.

National Association of Elementary School Principals, *Standards for quality elementary schools: School climate*. Reston, VA: Council for Exceptional Children.

National Association of Secondary School Principals, *School Climate Survey (Form A)*. Reston, VA: Council for Exceptional Children.

School Assessment Survey, Research for Better Schools. Philadelph ia, PA.

Sweeney, J. (1988). *Tips for improving school climate*. Arlington, VA: American Association of School Administrators.

Sweeney, J. *School Profile: Climate*. Ames, IA: Iowa State University.

Appendix C

References for the Enhancement of Self-Esteem

Albert, L. (1989). *A teacher's guide to cooperative discipline: How to manage your classroom and promote self-esteem*. Toronto, Ontario: Psycan.

Branden, N. (1985). *Honoring the self: The psychology of confidence and respect*. New York: Doubleday Dell.

Branden, N. (1988). *How to raise your self-esteem*. New York: Bantam.

Canfield, J. & Wells, H.C. (1976). *100 ways to enhance self-concept in the classroom: A handbook for teachers and parents*. Englewood, NJ: Prentice Hall.

Clemes, H., & Bean, R. (1981). *Self-esteem, the key to your child's well-being*. New York: Putman.

Coopersmith, S. (1967). *Antecedents of self-esteem*. San Francisco, CA: W.H. Freeman Company.

Frank, R.A., & Edwards, J.P. (1988). *Building self-esteem*: A guide for parents and professionals working with persons with developmental disabilities. Austin, TX: Pro-Ed.

Jose, R.T. (Ed.). (1983). Psychosocial aspects of low vision. In *Understanding low vision*. New York: American Foundation for the Blind.

Loumiet, R., & Levack, N. (1991). *Independent living: A curriculum with adaptations for students with visual impairments: Volume I: Social competence*. Austin, TX: Texas School for the Blind and Visually Impaired.

Mangold, S. (1980). Nurturing high self-esteem in visually handicapped children. In T.D. Yawley (Ed.), *The self concept of the young child*. Provo, UT: Brigham Young University.

Mangold, S. (1982). Nurturing high self-esteem in visually handicapped children. In S.S. Mangold (Ed.), *A teacher's guide to the special needs of blind and visually handicapped children*. New York: American Foundation for the Blind.

Mangold, S. (1988). Nurturing high self-esteem in adolescents with visual handicaps. *Journal of Vision Rehabilitation*, 2(3), 5-9.

McCabe, M.E., & Rhodes, J. (1988). *The nurturing classroom. Developing self-esteem, thinking skills and responsibility through simple cooperation*. Willits, CA: ITA Publications.

Reasoner, R.W., & Dusa, G.G. (1991). *Building self-esteemin the secondary schools: Teacher's manual*. Palo Alto, CA: The Cosulting Psychologist's Press.

Rousso, H. (1984). Fostering healthy self-esteem. *The Exceptional Parent, 14*(8), 11-17.

Tuttle, D.W. (1984). *Self-esteem and adjustment with blindness: The process of responding to life's demands*. Springfield, IL: Charles C. Thomas.

Walker, L.S., & Greene, J.W. (1986). The social context of adolescent self-esteem. *Journal of Youth and Adolescence, 15*(4), 315-322.

Walz, G.R., & Bleuer, J.C. (Eds.). (1992). *Student Self-Esteem A Vital Element of School Success*. Ann Arbor, MI: CAPS.

Resources on Self-Esteem

"Building Self-Esteem: A Comprehensive Program for Schools," Consulting Psychologists Press, 3803 E. Bayshore Road, Palo Alto, CA 94303

"Building Self-Esteem: A Guide for Parents, Schools, and Communities," a 27 page booklet published in 1991 by AASA, 1801 N. Moore St., Arlington, VA 22209

Tamaren, M.C. (1992). *I make a difference!: A curriculum guide building self-esteem and sensitivity in the inclusive classroom.* Novato, CA: Academic Therapy Publications.

Instruments for Assessing Self-Concept and Self-Esteem

Piers, E.V. (1984). *The Piers-Harris Children's Self-Concept Scale.* Los Angeles: Western Psychological Services.

Battle, J. (1980). *The Culture-Free Self-Esteem Inventories for Children and Adults.* Seattle: Special Publications.

Fitts, W.H. (1965). *The Tennessee Self-Concept Scale.* Los Angeles: Western Psychological Services.

Coppersmith, S. (1981). *The Coopersmith Self-Esteem Inventories.* Palo Alto, CA: Consulting Psychologi sts Press.

Rosenberg, M. (1979). The Rosenberg Self-Esteem Scale. In M. Rosenberg, Conceiving the self. New York: Basic Books .

Appendix D

Checklist of School Level Considerations

1. Integration perceived as significant innovation
2. Emphasis on the affective development of students
3. Promotion of development of student's self-esteem
4. Promotion of the positive acceptance of difference
5. Opportunity for adults to openly discuss their concerns relevant to integration
6. Identification and awareness of prejudices held and understanding of how these influence behaviour
7. Stated school philosophy relevant to integration of students with disabilities
8. Inclusion of all adults in the school in the discussion of philosophy and practice relevant to students with disabilities
9. Balance in curriculum between process and content
10. Balance in curriculum between affective and cognitive domains
11. Collaborative teams assigned to enhance social integration and positive acceptance of difference
12. Broad representation of staff, parents and students on collaborative teams
13. Principal's routine promotion of social integration
14. Formal plans to enhance, monitor and evaluate social integration
15. Meaningful teacher participation in the development and implementation of programs for students integrated in their classrooms
16. Meaningful parent participation in the development and implementation of programs for their child
17. Active participation of a trained teacher of the visually impaired to assist with the social acceptance and interaction of students who are visually impaired
18. Equally valued input from all members of the collaborative team
19. Problem-solving approach to analyzing and addressing social integration issues
20. Solutions generated to address social integration issues are specific to unique circumstances in the given school
21. Routine observation of student's interaction in various classes, activities and times of the year
22. Formal training in strategies to enhance the cognitive and affective development of students with disabilities for all teachers involved
23. Understanding of information and issues in the following areas:
    - philosophical, moral and practical issues inherent to integration
    - the nature and implications of visual impairment on learning and the development of social skills and the adaptations required to compensate for the lack of visual cues in interpersonal communication
    - awareness of pupil culture and implications for social integration of students with a disability
    - awareness of importance of childhood friendships and how they are negotiated
    - affective education and how to implement in the classroom
    - social skills and instruction in the classroom; and -strategies to promote the development of student self-esteem
24. Flexibility to experiment with various approaches to address the affective education needs of students

25. Educators trained in the methods of cooperative learning
26. Educators familiar with the use of assessment instruments designed to measure students' acceptance by peers, social skills, and level of self-esteem
27. Educators competent in assessing the social environment of schools and using information to plan strategies to enhance the social acceptance and interaction of students with disabilities
28. Educators and parents trained in effective observation of student behaviour in the classroom and on the playground.
29. Educators and parents who understand and promote the positive acceptance of difference

Checklist of Considerations Relevant to Students with a Visual Impairment

1. Commitment from all participants in social environment to realize goal of social integration
2. Social acceptance perceived as interdependent relationship between student with a visual impairment and her/his classmates
3. Availability of information obtained from formal and informal assessment of student with a visual impairment
4. Intervention based on assessment results, observation of student behaviour, and collective knowledge of collaborative team
5. Compulsory assessment of social skills
6. Social skills training programs incorporated in classroom instruction
7. Use of social skills training curriculum and resources designed specifically for students with a visual impairment in conjunction with generic programs
8. Routine assessment and monitoring of social skills
9. Involvement of students with a visual impairment in planning of social skills training
10. Use of a variety of instructional methods in teaching social skills
11. Analysis of social environment to determine factors which enhance and detract from social acceptance
12. Parent monitoring of practice of newly learned social skills in the home and community
13. Student understands visual impairment and its implications
14. Student encouraged to display self-initiative and self-advocacy
15. Student can generate solutions to problems of visual access
16. Student exposed to opportunities to discuss interests in common with peers
17. Plans for the meaningful involvement of student in all activities
18. Discouragement of the development of a special status associated with being visually impaired
19. Those unfamiliar with student with a visual impairment advised in advance of recommended approaches to use when interacting/working with the student
20. Difficulties or mistakes of adults routinely shared with students
21. Discouragement of practices which promote learned helplessness
22. Student responsible for initiating interaction with peers
23. Orchestration of opportunities for student to demonstrate competence
24. Opportunities for student to help others
25. Identification of organization skills which increase student's efficiency in the classroom

26. Student responsible for storage, retrieval and management of learning materials
27. Organization skills included in individual education program
28. Peers aware of problems nonverbal communication may create for those with a visual impairment
29. Acknowledgement of importance of accurate feedback on behaviour to student
30. Access to visual information both inside and outside the classroom
31. Identification of potential effects of visual impairment on development of high self-esteem
32. Monitoring of the subtle messages relevant to being visually impaired received by student
33. Availability of successful role models with a visual impairment
34. Display of positive images of persons with a visual impairment
35. Opportunities for student to spend time with other students with a visual impairment
36. Promotion of environment which emphasizes student's abilities and minimizes limitations imposed by visual impairment
37. Identification of realistic social and academic expectations for student
38. Involvement of parents in strategies to enhance high self-esteem
39. Absence of false praise
40. Encouragement used instead of praise
41. Feedback on student's behaviour/performance without judgement of character

Checklist of Considerations Relevant to Classmates of Student with a Visual Impairment

1. Involvement of classmates in promoting social integration
2. Classmates knowledgeable of visual impairment and its implications
3. Classmates generate solutions to social interaction problems
4. Classmates provide verbal feedback to student with visual impairment
5. Open discussion of visual impairment and its functional implications
6. Variety of strategies involving classmates in improving social integration of student with a visual impairment
7. Classmates provided special training in peer-based intervention strategies
8. Availability of peer support groups

References

Adams, M.J., & Faux, D.D. (1977). *Printing technology: A medium of visual communication*. Belmont, CA: Wadsworth Publishing Company.

Ainsworth, M.D.S. (1982). Attachment: Retrospect and prospect. In C.M. Parkes & J. Stevenson-Hinde (Eds.), *The place of attachment in human behavior*. New York: Basic Books.

Alfonso, R.J. (1986). *The unseen supervisor: Organization and culture as determinants of teacher behavior*. San Francisco, CA. (ERIC Document Reproduction Service No. ED 277 141)

Allport, G.W. (1958). *The nature of prejudice*. Garden City, NY: Doubleday Anchor Books.

Allport, G.W. (1980). Psychological problems of children with severely impaired vision. In B. Lowenfeld (Ed.), *Psychology of exceptional children*. New York: Prentice-Hall.

Ammerman, R.T., Van Hasselt, V.B., & Hersen, M. (1986). Psychological adjustment of visually handicapped children and youth. *Clinical Psychology Review, 6*, 67-85.

Andrews, J., & Lupart, J. (Eds.). (1993). *The inclusive classroom: Education exceptional children*. Scarborough, Ont: Nelson Canada.

Asher, S.R., & Gottman, J. (Ed.). (1981). *The development of children's friendships*. New York: Cambridge University Press.

Asher, S.R., & Taylor, A.R. (1981). Social outcomes of mainstreaming: Sociometric assessment and beyond. *Exceptional Educational Quarterly, 1*(4), 13-30.

Asher, S.R., Hymel, S., & Renshaw, P.D. (1984). Loneliness in children. *Childhood Development, 55*, 1456-1464.

Asher, S.R., Renshaw, P.D., & Hymel, S. (1982). Peer relations and the development of social skills. In S.G. Moore & C.R.

Cooper (Eds.), *The young child: Reviews of research* (Vol. 3). Washington, DC: National Association for the Education of Young Children.

Atlantic Provinces Special Education Authority. (1986). *Report of the study of off campus programs and services for hearing and visually impaired pupils*. Halifax, Nova Scotia.

Baker, L.D. (1973). Blindness and social behavior. *New Outlook for the Blind, 67*(7), 315-318.

Barraga, N. (1976). *Visual handicaps and learning: A developmental approach*. Belmont, CA: Wadsworth.

Barton, L. & Tomlinson, S. (Eds.). (1981). *Special education: Policy, practices and social issues*. London: Harper & Row.

Bee, H. (1989). *The developing child*. (5th ed.). New York: Harper & Row.

Bennett, B., Rolheiser-Bennett, C., & Stevahn, L. (1991). *Cooperative learning: Where heart meets mind*. Toronto: Ont: Educational Connections.

Berndt, T.J. (1982). The features and effects of friendship in early adolescence. *Child Development, 53*, 1447-1460.

Berndt, T. J. (1983). Social cognition, social behavior, and children's friendships. In E.T. Higgins, D.N. Ruble, & W.W. Hartup (Eds.), *Social cognition and social development: A sociocultural perspective*. New York: Cambridge University Press.

Biklen, D. (1985). *Achieving the complete school: Strategies for effective mainstreaming*. New York: Teachers College Press.

Bishop, V.E. (1986). Identifying the components of success in mainstreaming. *Journal of Visual Impairment and Blindness, 80*, 939-946.

Cairns, R.B. (1986). A contemporary perspective on social development. In P.S. Strain, M.J. Guralnick, & H.M. Walker (Eds.), *Children's social behavior: Development, assessment and modification*. Orlando, FL: Academic Press.

Chaffin, J.D. (1974). Will the real "mainstreaming" program please stand up! (or...should Dunn have done it?). *Focus on Exceptional Children, 6*(5), 3-17.

Chernus-Mansfield, N., Hayashi, D., Horn, M., & Kekelis, L.S. (1985). *Heart to heart: Parents of blind children talk about their feelings*. Los Angeles: Blind Childrens Center.

Chiu, L.H. (1992). Measure of self-esteem for school age children. In G. Walz & J. Bleuer, *Student self-esteem:*

A vital element of school success. Ann Arbor, MI: Counseling and Personal Services.

Cook-Clampert, D. (1981). The development of self-concept in blind children. *Journal of Visual Impairment and Blindness, 75*(5), 233-238.

Corn, A.L. (1985). An independence matrix for visually impaired learners. *Education of the Visually Handicapped, 18*(1), 3-10.

Corn, A.L. (1987). Socialization and the child with low vision. *Proceedings of the Sixth Interdisciplinary Symposium on the Visually Impaired Child* (pp. 21-46). Halifax, Nova Scotia.

Corn, A., & Bishop, V.E. (1984). Acquisition of practical knowledge by blind and visually impaired students in grades 8-12. *Journal of Visual Impairment and Blindness, 78*, 352-356.

Corsaro, W.A. (1981). Friendship in the nursery school: Social organization in a peer environment. In S. Asher & J. Gottman (Eds.), *The development of children's friendships*. Cambridge: Cambridge University Press.

Corsaro, W.A. (1985). *Friendship and peer culture in the early years*. Norwood, NJ: Ablex.

Cowen, E.L., Pederson, A., Babigian, H., Izzo, L.D., & Trost, M.A. (1973). Long-term follow-up of early detected vulnerable children. *Journal of Consulting and Clinical Psychology, 41*, 438-446.

Crandell, J.M., & Streeter, L. (1977). The social adjustment of blind students in different educational settings. *Education of the Visually Handicapped*, 9(1), 1-7.

Curry, S.A., & Hatlen, P.H. (1988). Meeting the unique educational needs of visually impaired pupils through appropriate placement. *Journal of Visual Impairment and Blindness, 82*), 417-424.

Czerwinski, M., & Tait, P. (1981). Blind children's perception of normal, withdrawn and antisocial behavior. *Journal of Visual Impairment and Blindness, 75*, 252-257.

Dahl, H. (1986). The education of severely and profoundly handicapped children and youth: Some issues that currently need to be resolved. *Proceedings of the Canadian Symposium on Special Education Issues*. (C, 1-14). Toronto: The Ontario Council of Administrators of Special Education.

Davidson, I. & Nesker Simmons, J. (Eds.). (1992). *The early development of blind children: A book of readings*. Toronto, ONT: OISE Press.

Davies, B. (1982). *Life in the classroom and playground: The accounts of primary school children*. Boston: Routledge and Kegan Paul.

Davies, B. (1984). Friends and fights. In M. Hammersley and P. Woods (Eds.), *Life in school*. Milton Keynes: Open University Press.

Davis, F. (1961). Deviance disavowal: The management of strained interaction by the visibly handicapped. *Social Problems, 9*, 120-132.

Delamont, S. (Ed.). (1984). *Reading on interaction in the classroom*. London: Methuen.

DePauw, K. (1981). Physical education for the visually impaired: Review of the literature. *Journal of Visual Impairment and Blindness*, *75*, 162-164.

Dodge, K.A. (1983). Behavioral antecedents of peer social status. *Child Development, 54*, 1386-1399.

Eaglestein, A.S. (1975). The social acceptance of blind high school students in an integrated setting. *New Outlook for the Blind, 69*, 447-451.

Epstein, J.L. (1986). Friendship selection: Developmental and environmental influences. In E.C. Mueller & C.R. Cooper (Eds.), *Process and outcome in peer relationships*. New York: Academic Press.

Forest, M., Vandercook, T., & York, J. (1989). The McGill Action Plann ing Syste m (MAPS): A strategy for building the vision. Journal of the Association for Persons with Severe Handicaps, *14*, 205-215.

Fine, G.A. (1981). Friends, impression management, and preadolescent behavior. In S.R. Asher & J.M. Gottman (Eds.), *The development of children's friendships*. Cambridge: Cambridge University Press.

Fraiberg, S. (1977). *Insights from the blind: Comparative studies of blind and sighted infants*. New York: Basic Books.

Frank, R.A., & Edwards, J.P. (1988). *Building self-esteem: A guide for parents and professionals working with persons with developmental disabilities*. Austin, TX: Pro-Ed.

Fundis, A.T. (1981). Social interaction with peers: A developmental perspective on social isolation. *Exceptional Educational Quarterly*, *1*(4), 1-12.

Gall, R.S. (1987). Framework for policy and action in special education: An international perspective. In *The future of special education: Proceedings of the CEC Symposium*. Reston, VA: Council for Exceptional Children.

Gaylord-Ross, R. (Ed.). (1989). *Integration strategies for students with handicaps*. Baltimore, MD: Paul H. Brookes Publishing.

Glasser, W. (1969). *Schools without failure*. New York: Harper and Row.

Gottman, J.M. (1976). Stage development of blind children: A Piagetian view. *New Outlook for the Blind, 70*, 94-100.

Gottman, J.M. & Parker, J.G. (1986). *Conversations of friends*. Cambridge, MA: Cambridge Press.

Goupil, G., & Comeau, M. (1983). Le statut sociometrique des eleves handicapes de la vue integres dans les classes regulieres du Quebec. *Canadian Journal of Education, 8*, 362-372.

Gresham, F.M. (1982). Misguided mainstreaming: The case for social skills training with handicapped children. *Exceptional Children, 48*, 422-433.

Gresham, F.M. (1983). Social skills assessment as a component of mainstreaming placement decisions. *Exceptional Children, 49*, 331-336.

Guralnick, M.J. (1981). Programming factors affecting child-child social interactions in mainstreamed preschool programs. *Exceptional Education Quarterly*, *1*, 71-92.

Hallinan, M.T., & Smith, S.S. (1987). *Classroom characteristics and student friendship cliques*. Bethesda, MD: National Institute of Child Health and Human Development. (ERIC Document Reproduction Service No. ED 280 611)

Hamilton, S.F. (1983). The social side of schooling: Ecological studies of classrooms and schools. *The Elementary School Journal, 83*(4), 313-334.

Hammersley, M., & Woods, P. (Eds.). (1984). *Life in school: The sociology of pupil culture*. Milton Keynes: Open University Press.

Hargreaves, D.H. (1975). Interpersonal relations and education. London: Routledge & Kegan Paul.

Harrell, R.L., & Strauss, F.A. (1986). Approaches to increasing assertive behavior and communication skills in blind and visually impaired persons. *Journal of Visual Impairment and Blindness, 80*, 794-798.

Harris, W. (1984). *Making better choices: A curriculum for teaching cognitive planning and social skills to improve social and academic behavior*. Oreno, ME: University of Maine.

Hartup, W.W. (1984). The peer context in middle childhood. In W.A. Collins (Ed.), *Development during middle childhood*. Washington, D.C.: National Academic Press.

Hatlen, P.H., & Curry, S.A. (1987). In support of specialized programs for blind and visually impaired children: The impact of vision loss on learning. *Journal of Visual Impairment and Blindness, 81*, 7-13.

Hinde, R.A., & Stevenson-Hinde, J. (1987). Interpersonal relationships and child development. *Developmental Review, 7*, 1-21.

Hoben, M. (1976). *Reducing Isolation in the Mainstream: Final Report*. Minneapolis: Hennepin Technical Centers.

Hoben, M. (1979). *Integration of visually impaired students and hearing impaired students in regular classrooms: A report of research*. Hennepin Technical Centers, Minneapolis, MN. (ERIC Document Reproduction Service No. 177 839)

Hoben, M. (1980). Toward integration in the mainstream. *Exceptional Children, 47,* 100-105.

Hoben, M. & Lindstom, V. (1980). Evidence of isolation in the mainstream. *Journal of Visual Impairment and Blindness, 74*, 289-292.

Huebner, K. (1986). Social skills. In G.Scholl (Ed.), *Foundations of education for blind and visually handicapped children and youth: Theory and practice*. New York: American Foundation for the Blind.

Hull, W. (1983). Social development of preschool visually handicapped children. In M.E. Mulholland & M.V. Wurster (Eds.), *Help me become everything I can be*. New York: American Foundation for the Blind.

Hurt, H.T., Scott, M.D., & McCroskey, J.C. (1978). *Communication in the classroom*. Reading, MA: Addison-Wesley.

Johnson, D.W. & Johnson, R.T. (1989). *Leading the cooperative school*. Edina, MN: Interaction Book.

Johnson, D.W., Johnson, R.T. & Holubec, E.J. (1987). *Structuring cooperative learning: Lesson plans for teachers*. Edina, MN: Interaction Book.

Johnson, D.W., Johnson, R.T. & Holubec, E.J. (1990). *Circles of learning: Cooperation in the classroom*. Edina, MN: Interaction Book.

Johnson, D.W., Johnson, R.T. & Holubec, E.J. (1991). *Cooperation in the classroom*. Edina, MN: Interaction Book Company.

Johnson, D.W., & Johnson, R.T. (1980). Integrating handicapped students into the mainstream. *Exceptional Children, 47*(2), 90-98.

Johnson, R.T., & Johnson, D.W. (1981). Building friendships between handicapped and non-handicapped children: Effects of cooperative and individualistic instruction. *American Educational Research Journal, 18*, 415-423.

Johnson, R.T., & Johnson, D.W. (1984). Classroom learning structure and attitudes toward handicapped students in mainstream settings: A theoretical model and research evidence. In R.L. Jones (Ed.), *Attitudes and attitude change in special education: Theory and practice*. Reston, VA: Council for Exceptional Children.

Jones, R.L., & Chiba, C. (1985). *Social skills assessment and intervention (Final Report)*. Bethesda, MD: National Institute of Child Health and Human Development.

Jones, R.L., Lavine, K., & Shell, J. (1972). Blind children integrated in classrooms with sighted children. *New Outlook for the Blind, 66*(3), 75-80.

Jose, R.T. (Ed.). (1983). Psychosocial aspects of low vision. In *Understanding low vision*. New York: American Foundation for the Blind.

Kirchner, C. (1990). Trends in the prevalence rates and numbers of blind and visually impaired schoolchildren. *Journal of Visual Impairment and Blindness, 84*, 478-479.

Kurdek, L.A., & Krile, D. (1982). A developmentaly analysis of the relationship between peer acceptance and both interpersonal understanding and perceived social competence. *Child Development, 53*, 1485-1491.

Lindley, L. (1990). Defining TASH: A mission statement. *TASH Newsletter, 16*(8), #1.

Loumiet, R. & Levack, N. (1991). *Independent Living: A curriculum with adaptations for students with visual impairments*. Austin, TX: Texas School for the Blind.

Lowenfeld, B. (1975). *The Changing Status of the Blind*. Springfield, IL: Charles C. Thomas.

Lowenfeld, B. (1980). Psychological problems of children with impaired vision. In W.N. Cruickshank (Ed.), *The psychology of exceptional children and youth*. Englewood Cliffs, N.J.: Prentice Hall.

MacCuspie, P.A. (1991). *The social acceptance and interaction of integrated visually impaired children*. Unpublished doctoral thesis. Halifax, N.S.: Dalhousie University.

MacCuspie, P.A. (1992). The social acceptance and interaction of visually impaired children in integrated settings. In S. Sacks, L.S. Kekelis & R. Gaylord-Ross (Eds.). *The development of social skills by blind and visually impaired students*. New York: American Foundation for the Blind.

MacCuspie, P.A., Harmer, D., McConnell, J., Fricker, J., & Johnson, J. (1993). Short-term placements : A critical role for residential schools. *Journal of Visual Impairment and Blindness, 87*, 193-198.

MacCuspie, P.A., (1993). The responsibility of educators to facilitate social skills development in the school environment. *Proceedings of Eighth International Conference on Blind and Visually Impaired Children*, (111-121). Edmonton, AL: The Canadian National Institute for the Blind

MacCuspie, P.A., (1993). Development of social skills in children with a visual impairment : Strategies and practices. *Proceedings of Eighth International Conference on Blind and Visually Impaired Children*, (121-152). Edmonton, AL: The Canadian National Institute for the Blind.

MacFarland, D. (1966). Social isolation of the blind: An underrated aspect of disability and dependency. *New Outlook for the Blind, 60*, 318-319.

MacKay, W.A. (1986). The charter of rights and special education: Blessing or curse? *Proceedings of the Canadian Symposium on Special Education Issues*, (E, 1-30). Toronto: The Ontario Council of Administrators of Special Education.

MacMillan, D., & Morrison, G.M. (1984). Sociometric research in special education. In R.L. Jones (Ed.), *Attitudes and attitude change in special education: Theory and practice*. Reston, VA: Council for Exceptional Children.

Mangold, S. (1980). Nurturing high self-esteem in visually handicapped children. In T.D. Yawley (Ed.), *The self concept of the young child*. Provo, UT: Brigham Young University.

Mangold, S. (1982). Nurturing high self-esteem in visually handicapped children. In S.S. Mangold (Ed.), *A teacher's guide to the special needs of blind and visually handicapped children*. New York: American Foundation for the Blind.

Mangold, S. (1988). Nurturing high self-esteem in adolescents with visual handicaps. *Journal of Vision Rehabilitation*, 2(3), 5-9.

Matsuda, M.M. (1984). A comparative analysis of blind and sighted children's communication skills. *Journal of Visual Impairment and Blindness, 78,* 1-5.

Mayadas, N.S., & Duehn, W.D. (1976). The impact of significant adults' expectations on the life style of visually impaired children. *New Outlook for the Blind, 70,* 286-290.

McAlpine, L. (1992). *The developing social understanding in visually impaired children*. Unpublished paper. Halifax, N.S.: Dalhousie University

McCabe, M.E., & Rhodes, J. (1988). *The nurturing classroom. Developing self-esteem, thinking skills and responsibility through simple cooperation*. Willits, CA: ITA Publications.

Mead, G. (1934). *Mind, self, and society*. Chicago: University of Chicago Press.

Mehan, H. (1978). Structuring school structure. *Harvard Educational Review, 48*(1), 32-64.

Meyers, C., MacMillan, D., & Yoshida, R. (1980). Regular class education of EMR students, from efficacy to mainstreaming: A review of issues and research. In J. Gottlieb (Ed.), *Educating mentally retarded persons in the mainstream*. Baltimore: University Park Press.

Minter, M.E., Hobson, R.P., & Pring, L. (1991). Recognition of vocally expressed emotion by congenitally blind children. *Journal of Visual Impairment and Blindness, 85,* 411-415.

Monbeck, M.E. (1975). *The meaning of blindness*. Bloomington, IN: Indiana University Press.

Morse, J. (1983). Psychological aspects of low vision. In R.T. Jose (Ed.). *Understanding low vision*. New York: American Foundation for the Blind.

Morse, W.C., Ardizzone, J., Macdonald, C., & Pasick, P. (1980). *Affective education for special children and youth*. Reston, VA: The Council for Exceptional Children.

New Brunswick Department of Education. (1994). *Teacher assistant guidelines for standards and evaluation*, Student Services Branch. Fredericton, New Brunswick.

Nesker Simmons, J., & Davidson, I. (1992). *Determinates of development: Conceptualizing young blind children*. Toronto, ONT: Ontario Institute of Studies in Education.

Nezer, H., Nezer, B., & Siperstein, G. (1985). *Improving children's social skills: Techniques for teachers* (Grant # DIE G5583016). Boston, MA: The Center for the Study of Social Acceptance, University of Massachusetts.

Nixon, H. (1991). *Mainstreaming and the American dream: Sociological perceptions on parental coping with blind and visually impaired children*. New York: American Foundation for the Blind.

Olson, M. (1986). Stereotypic mannerisms of visually handicapped children. *DVH Quarterly, 30(2)*, 14-19.

Orlick, T. (1978). *The cooperative sports and games book*. New York: Pantheon.

Orlick, T. (1978a). *Winning through cooperation*. Washington, D.C.: Acropolis.

Orlick, T. (1981). *The second cooperative sports and games book*. New York: Pantheon.

Parker, J.G., & Asher, S.R. (1987). Peer relations and later adjustment: Are low-accepted children "at risk"? *Psychological Bulletin, 102*, 357-389.

Parsons, S. (1986a). Functions of play in low vision children. Part I. *Journal of Visual Impairment and Blindness, 80*, 627-630.

Parsons, S. (1986b). Functions of play in low vision children. Part II. *Journal of Visual Impairment and Blindness, 80*, 777-784.

Parsons, S. (1987). Locus of control and adaptive behavior in visually impaired children. *Journal of Visual Impairment and Blindness, 81*, 429-432.

Piaget, J. (1973). *The child and reality*. New York: Grossman.

Pollard, A. (1985). *The social world of the primary school*. Eastbourne, East Sussex: Holt, Rinehart, & Winston.

Purkey, S., & Smith, M. (1982). "Too soon to cheer? Synthesis on research on effective schools". *Educational Leadership, 39*, 64-69.

Quintal, J. (1986). How are we doing? Issues and research related to the integration of students with special needs. *Proceedings of the Canadian Symposium on Special Education Issues,* (A,1-13). Toronto, ONT: The Ontario Council of Administrators of Special Education.

Raver, S. (1986). *Training gaze direction in blind children: Attitude effects on the sighted*. Paper presented at the annual convention of the Council for Exceptional Children, New Orleans, LA. (Eric Document Reproduction Service No. Ed. 268 756)

Raver, S.A. & Drash, P.W. (1988). Increasing social skills training for visually impaired children. *Education of the Visually Handicapped, 19*, 147-155.

Reynolds, M. (1976). Mainstreaming: Historical perspectives. In P.A. O'Donnell, & R.H. Bradfield (Eds.), *Mainstreaming: Controversy and consensus*. San Rafael, CA: Academic Therapy.

Reynolds, M.C. (1983). The new surge for mainstreaming. In M.E. Mulholland & M.V. Wurster (Eds.), *Help me become everything I can be*. New York: American Foundation for the Blind.

Reynolds, M., Wang, M., & Walberg, H. (1987). The necessary restructuring of special and regular education. *Exceptional Children, 53*, 391-397.

Robinson, G., Jan, J. & Kinnis, C. (1987). Congenital ocular blindness in children, 1945 to 1984. *American Journal of Diseases of Children, 141*, 1321-1324.

Rogers, C. (1982). *A social psychology of schooling: The expectancy process*. London: Routledge and Kegan Paul.

Rogow, S. (1988). *Helping the visually impaired child with developmental problems*. New York: Teachers College Press.

Rubin, K.H., & Ross, H.S. (Eds.). (1982). *Peer relationship and social skills in childhood*. New York: Springer-Verlag.

Rubin, Z. (1980). *Children's friendships*. London: Fontana.

Sabornie, E.J. (1985). Social mainstreaming of handicapped students: Facing an unpleasant reality. *Remedial and Special Education, 6*, 12-16.

Sacks, S., Kekelis, L.S. & Gaylord-Ross, R.J. (Eds.). (1992) *The development of social skills by blind and visually impaired students*. New York: American Foundation for the Blind.

Sacks, S., & Reardon, M.P. (1989). Maximizing social interaction for students with visual handicaps. In R. Gaylord-Ross (Ed.), *Integration strategies for students with handicaps*. Baltimore, MD: Paul H. Brookes.

Salvia, J. & Ysseldyke, J. (1991). *Assessment*. (5th Edition). Boston, MA: Houghton Mifflin.

Santin, S., & Simmons, J.N. (1977). Problems in the construction of reality of congenitally blind children. *Journal of Visual Impairment and Blindness, 71*, 425-429.

Sapon-Shevin, M. (1978). Another look at mainstreaming: Exceptionality, normality, and the nature of difference. *Phi Delta Kappan, 60*(2), 119-121.

Schein, E.H. (1985). *Organizational culture and leadership*. San Francisco: Jossey-Bass.

Scholl, G. (Ed.). (1986). *Foundations of education for blind and visually handicapped children and youth: Theory and practice*. New York: American Foundation for the Blind.

Scott, R.A. (1969a). The socialization of blind children. In D.A. Goslin (Ed.), *Handbook of socialization theory and research*. Chicago: Rand McNally & Co.

Scott, R.A. (1969b). *The making of blind men: A study of adult socialization*. New York: Russell Sage Foundation.

Sergiovanni, T.J. (1984). Leadership and excellence in schooling. *Educational Leadership, 41*(5), 4-13.

Shea, T.M., & Bauer, A.M. (1994). *Learners with disabilities: A social systems perspective of special education*. Madison,WI: WCB Brown & Benchmark.

Sieber, R.T. (1979a). Classmates as workmates: Informal peer activity in the elementary school. *Anthropology and Education Quarterly, 10*, 207-235.

Sieber, R.T. (1979b). Schoolrooms, pupils, and rules: The role of informality in bureaucratic socialization. *Human Organization, 38*, 273-282.

Sieber. R.T. (1981). *Children and their organizations: Investigations in American culture*. Boston: Hall.

Skrtic, T. (1987). *An organizational analysis of special education reform*. Lawrence, KS: University of Kansas.

Smith, T.E.C., & Smith, B.L. (1983). Using participant observation to determine the social behaviour of visually handicapped children. *Education of the Visually Handicapped, 15*(1), 30-36.

Sonksen, P.M. (1983). Vision and early development. In K. Wybar & D. Taylor (Eds.), *Pediatric Ophthalmology: Current Aspects*. New York: Marcell Dekker.

Spender, D. (1982). *Invisible women: The schooling scandal*. London: Writers and Readers.

Stain, P.S., Guralnick, M.J., & Walker, H.M. (Eds.). (1986). Children's social behavior: Development, assessment, and modification. Orlando, FL: Academic Press.

Sullivan, K. (1989). *Multicultural assumptions of selected school boards in Nova Scotia*. Halifax, N.S.: Dalhousie University.

Swallow, R. M., & Huebner, K.M. (Eds.). (1987). *How to thrive not just survive: A guide to developing independent life skills for blind and visually impaired children and youth*. New York: American Foundation for the Blind.

Sweeney, J. (1988). *Tips for improving school climate*. Arlington, VA: American Association of School Administrators.

Tuttle, D.W. (1984). *Self-esteem and adjustment with blindness: The process of responding to life's demands*. Springfield,IL: Charles C. Thomas.

Vander Kolk, C.V., & Bright, B.C. (1983). Albinism: A survey of attitudes and behavior. *Journal of Visual Impairment and Blindness, 77*, 49-51.

Van Hasselt, V.B., Simon, J., & Mastantuono, A.K. (1982). Social skills training for blind children and adolescents. *Education of the Visually Handicapped, 14*(2), 34-39.

Van Hasselt, V.B. (1983). Social adaptation in the blind. *Clinical Psychology Review, 3*, 87-102.

Vickers, R. (1987). A psychological approach to attitudes toward blind persons. *Journal of Visual Impairment and Blindness, 81*(7), 323-325.

Voeltz, L. M. (1984). Program and curriculum innovations to prepare children for integration. In N. Certo, N. Haring & R. York (Eds.), *Public school integration of severely handicapped students*. Baltimore, MD: Paul H. Brooks

Walker, L.S., & Greene, J.W. (1986). The social context of adolescent self-esteem. *Journal of Youth and Adolescence, 15*(4), 315-322.

Walz, G.R., & Bleuer, J.C. (Eds.). (1992). *Student self-esteem: A Vital Element of School Success*. Ann Arbor , MI: CAPS.

Warren, D.H. (1984). *Blindness and early childhood development* (2nd ed.). New York: American Foundation for the Blind.

Winzer, M. (1990). *Children with exceptionalities: A Canadian perspective*. Scarborough, ONT: Prentice-Hall.

Winzer, M., Rogow, S., & David, C. (1987). *Exceptional children in Canada*. Scarborough, Ontario: Prentice-Hall.

Wolfensberger, W. (1972). *The principal of normalization in human services*. Toronto: National Institute on Mental Retardation.

Woods, P. (1979). *The divided school*. London: Routledge & Kegan Paul.

Woods, P. (1980). *Pupil strategies*. London: Croom Helm.

Woods, P. (1983). *Sociology and the school*. London: Routledge and Kegan Paul.

Workman, S.H. (1986). Teachers' verbalizations and the social interaction of blind preschoolers. *Journal of Visual Impairment and Blindness, 80*, 532-534.